New Directions in Cultural Policy Research

Series Editor
Eleonora Belfiore, Department of Social Sciences, Loughborough University, Loughborough, UK

New Directions in Cultural Policy Research encourages theoretical and empirical contributions which enrich and develop the field of cultural policy studies. Since its emergence in the 1990s in Australia and the United Kingdom and its eventual diffusion in Europe, the academic field of cultural policy studies has expanded globally as the arts and popular culture have been re-positioned by city, regional, and national governments, and international bodies, from the margins to the centre of social and economic development in both rhetoric and practice. The series invites contributions in all of the following: arts policies, the politics of culture, cultural industries policies (the 'traditional' arts such as performing and visual arts, crafts), creative industries policies (digital, social media, broadcasting and film, and advertising), urban regeneration and urban cultural policies, regional cultural policies, the politics of cultural and creative labour, the production and consumption of popular culture, arts education policies, cultural heritage and tourism policies, and the history and politics of media and communications policies. The series will reflect current and emerging concerns of the field such as, for example, cultural value, community cultural development, cultural diversity, cultural sustainability, lifestyle culture and eco-culture, planning for the intercultural city, cultural planning, and cultural citizenship.

Molly Mullen · Rand Hazou · Sarah Woodland
Editors

Artful Evaluation for Creative Health and Wellbeing

palgrave
macmillan

Editors
Molly Mullen
University of Auckland
Auckland, New Zealand

Rand Hazou
Massey University
Auckland, New Zealand

Sarah Woodland
University of Melbourne
Melbourne, VIC, Australia

ISSN 2730-924X ISSN 2730-9258 (electronic)
New Directions in Cultural Policy Research
ISBN 978-3-032-17062-0 ISBN 978-3-032-17063-7 (eBook)
https://doi.org/10.1007/978-3-032-17063-7

This work was supported by University of Auckland.

Cover illustration: Jeanne Leclercq

This Palgrave Macmillan imprint is published by the registered company Springer Nature Switzerland AG
The registered company address is: Gewerbestrasse 11, 6330 Cham, Switzerland

Foreword: Measuring What Matters

How do we measure a "spring in the step" or a "gleam in the eye"? How do we trace the subtle shifts that occur when someone finds their voice, reclaims a story, or feels, perhaps for the first time, truly seen?

Emerging from the *Precarity, Creative Arts, and Wellbeing Symposium* held in Aotearoa New Zealand, *Artful Evaluation* does not pretend to offer neat answers. Instead, it extends an invitation—generous, grounded, and bold. It calls us to reimagine what counts as knowledge, how value is created, and who gets to decide. The book reminds us that evaluation, at its best, is not a tool to pass judgement but a relationship to which all are accountable. It is not a measuring stick, but a form of witnessing.

The stories collected in these pages give space to those too often written out of dominant narratives. They centre the philosophical play of learning-disabled artists in, for example, the quiet intimacy of voice-note exchanges among those living with Long COVID, and the complex presence of grief, resistance, and joy within communities navigating systemic harm. These works do not seek validation through traditional metrics alone. Instead, they offer new meanings that are rooted in care, co-presence, cultural specificity, and radical attentiveness.

A through-line in this collection is the call for *epistemic justice* to centre ways of knowing that have been marginalised, dismissed, or pathologised. Who gets to produce knowledge? Who is listened to? And what does it mean to listen well? How do we value *art* and why do we value *usefulness*?

Artful Evaluation answers that call with clarity and care. In this volume, the answer lies in Indigenous-led methodologies, in feminist and decolonial frameworks, and in the everyday artistry of community practitioners who disrupt binaries between rigour and resonance, evidence and experience, method and meaning. In a world marked by the aftershocks of a global pandemic, widening social divides, and the slow violence of ecological collapse, this book offers practices not only for reflection, but for repair. Across regions and disciplines, a shared imperative is emerging: to develop evaluation practices that are locally rooted, culturally responsive, and ethically attuned—an imperative echoed in foundational works such as Linda Tuhiwai Smith's (1999) *Decolonizing Methodologies* and Sarah Ahmed's (2019) *On the Uses of Use*, upon which this text builds.

This collection reflects the vibrancy and complexity of creative health practice in Aotearoa and Australia, while also offering globally resonant frameworks—ways of noticing, listening, and accounting for the relational, affective, and ecological dimensions of participatory arts, especially in contexts marked by precarity, marginalisation, and ongoing transformation. At the same time, the authors do not romanticise the arts. They remain keenly aware of power—of tokenism masquerading as co-design, of lived experience harvested for impact metrics. Their gaze is clear-eyed, and yet hopeful. This is not a utopian imagining. It is a careful stitching-together of practices that honour contradiction, embrace ambiguity, and make space for the not-yet-known.

References to the *Peckham Experiment*, in which lead researchers reflected on vital markers of health glimpsed in a sparkle, a gesture, a shift in posture, return like a refrain. These subtle signals—the quickening of spirit, the softening of breath, the lift in someone's gaze—are offered as data of a different kind. They do not fit easily into spreadsheets, but they speak clearly in the language of presence and aliveness. They are signs that something meaningful has occurred—signs best communicated through film, photography, theatre, and choreography.

Artful Evaluation is for artists, facilitators, health workers, researchers, policymakers, and all who recognise that culture and care are not separate spheres but entangled commitments. It is for those disillusioned by rigid dashboards, those interested in mixed methods and arts-based research, and those moved by the invisible architectures of healing, relationship, and co-creation. Here, evaluation is not about justification—it is about justice.

Nisha Sajnani
PhD, Associate Professor
and Director, Program in Drama
Therapy and Theatre and Health
Lab, Co-Director, Jameel Arts &
Health Lab
NYU Steinhardt
New York, NY, USA

Mauricio Salgado
MFA, Chair, Department
of Drama
NYU Tisch
New York, NY, USA

Nisha Sajnani PhD., RDT-BCT is the Director of the Program in Drama Therapy and Theatre & Health Lab; founder of the Arts & Health @NYU; and Chair of the NYU Creative Arts Therapies Consortium. In her capacity as founding co-director of the Jameel Arts & Health Lab, established in collaboration with the WHO to measurably improve health and wellbeing through the arts, Dr. Sajnani leads a *Lancet* global series on the health benefits of the arts. An award-winning author, educator, and advocate, her body of work explores the unique ways in which aesthetic experience can inspire equity, care, and collective human flourishing across the lifespan.

Mauricio Salgado is an Assistant Arts Professor of Theatre Studies, Director of Applied Theatre, and the Associate Chair in the Department of Drama. Mauricio is mestizo + first gen + born to proudly subversive Colombians + brown skinned + amateur bio-regionalist + aspiring theologian + cis-hetero + married + father + artist, pursuing justice and healing through a decolonial framework. He collaborates to organise space where folx rehearse revolution, compromise, rage, tolerance, strength, trust, and vulnerability. Prior to joining Tisch Drama, Salgado co-founded Arts Ignite (Formerly ASTEP). At Arts Ignite, he recruited, trained, and supported more than 325 teaching artists and created and implemented 23 programmes for artistic youth.

Acknowledgements

It takes a village to raise a child, and, perhaps also to produce a book. This volume is testament to the creative energies and critical rigour of a whole host of communities who have inspired this book's development. We would particularly like to acknowledge contributions and discussions facilitated by our research and artistic networks including Te Ora Auaha: Creative Wellbeing Alliance Aotearoa, and the Arts and Wellbeing Research and Evaluation Network (Aotearoa NZ and Australia). These networks prepared the ground and advanced considerations of creative health and wellbeing out of which this book emerged.

We would like to thank the keynotes and participants of the "Precarity, Creative Arts, and Wellbeing Symposium" which was co-convened at Massey University in Auckland in September 2023. These included keynotes by Shiloh Groot, Fran Kewene, Ying Wang, and Adrian Jackson whose presentations inspired further discussion and engagements that also inspired the development of this book.

We acknowledge the funding received from Waipapa Taumata Rau—the University of Auckland's Faculty of Education and Social Work's Research Development Grant. These funds enabled us to make the book Open Access and to resource the participation of chapter collaborators who work outside academia.

Contents

1 **Introduction: Re-evaluating Evaluation** 1
Molly Mullen, Sarah Woodland, and Rand Hazou

Part I What is of Value

2 **What Is of Value in the Learning Disabled Theatre of Different Light?** 31
Tony McCaffrey

3 **Southside Stories: Pacific Artists, Funding, Evaluation and Wellbeing in South Auckland** 51
Michelle Johansson

Part II Justice-Oriented Evaluation

4 **Queevaluing The Coming Back Out Ball: Towards a Creative Framework of Self-Determined Values** 73
Peta Murray, Marnie Badham, Tristan Meecham, and Bec Reid

5 **Home Ground: Evaluating in the Liminal Space** 93
Jacqui Moyes and Fran Kewene

6 **Listening, Witnessing, and Creative Repair: Towards Justice-Oriented Approaches to Valuing Lived Experience Expertise and Trauma-Informed Co-creative Practice** 113
Poppy de Souza and Rebecca J. Moran

Part III Community Wellbeing, Participation and Self-Determination

7 **Experimenting with Life in Vacant Spaces: Reflections on Assessing and Communicating Holistic Wellbeing Outcomes** 133
Kelly Dombroski

8 **Hobson Street Theatre Company: Developing an Evaluation Framework** 155
Rand Hazou, Bronwyn Bent, Joeli Thacker, John Hughes, Richard Nightingale, Leonard Mathews, Kelly Tunui, and Gem McIver

9 **Project X: Co-Creating a Meaningful Evaluation Framework for a Creative Youth Wellbeing Programme in Aotearoa** 173
Amber Walls and Borni Te Rongopai Tukiwaho

10 **Participatory Songwriting as Evaluative Research: Learning from Adolescent Experiences of Voice and Voicelessness** 195
Gillian Howell

Part IV Arts as Evaluative Practices

11 **Contested Zones: Circus Science Collaboration on Issues of Australian Ecologies** 219
Linda Hassall and Natalie Lazaroo

12 **Fleshy Socialities: Evaluative Practices in Theatre, Performance, Health, and Wellbeing** 241
Molly Mullen, Kelly Freebody, Kim Snider, and Elise Sterback

13 Conclusion 261
Rand Hazou, Sarah Woodland, and Molly Mullen

Index 267

Notes on Contributors

Marnie Badham has a 25-year history of art and justice practice in both Canada and Australia. Marnie's creative and critical research sits at the intersection of socially engaged art practice, participatory advocacy research methodologies, and the politics of cultural measurement. Through aesthetic and dialogic forms of encounter and exchange, Marnie's collaborative social practices bring together disparate groups of people (artists, communities, industry, local government) in dialogue to examine and affect local issues. Marnie is Associate Professor at RMIT University in Naarm/Melbourne.

Poppy de Souza is an interdisciplinary researcher and cultural practitioner whose work leans across cultural, creative, and critical research and practice. She is currently Postdoctoral Research Fellow with the Big Anxiety Research Centre (BARC), University of New South Wales, Sydney. Poppy's scholarship critically analyses the politics of voice and listening in conditions of inequality and injustice at border and threshold sites with a focus on sites and practices of struggle, resistance, and transformation. Her work has explored the relationship between sound, race, and (in)justice; and sonic, sensory, and embodied methods of listening and attunement. With Emma Russell, Poppy is also working on a book project, titled Sensing the Carceral State.

Different Light Theatre is an ensemble of learning-disabled artists. The company has been devising, performing, and researching performance for nineteen years in New Zealand. They have toured performances to Australia, the United States, and the UK, and members of the group have recently participated in online performance conferences in Athens, Helsinki, and Reykjavik.

Kelly Dombroski is an Associate Professor in Geography at Massey University (Palmerston North) and a Rutherford Discovery Fellow of Te Aparangi Royal Society of New Zealand. Over the last decade, her research has been focused on community economies in Aotearoa and Asia-Pacific more broadly. She has previously served on the board of Life in Vacant Spaces and is a current board member of the Community Economies Institute. She is Tangata Tiriti and lived and worked in Christchurch from 2013 to 2022.

Kelly Freebody is an Associate Professor in the Faculty of Arts and Social Sciences, the University of Sydney. Her research work merges her key interests in education, drama, social justice, youth, and community relationships. Her programme of research seeks to develop theoretical and practical understandings of the ways in which drama of/for/about social justice operates in a variety of institutional and educational settings. Using innovative methodologies drawn from the fields of critical policy studies, interaction analyses, sociology, and education, her work aims to provide new perspectives for researchers and practitioners in theatre, drama education, and school and community education. Kelly teaches in the Secondary Education programme on core units exploring pedagogy, educational policy enactment, educational sociology, creativity, and drama/theatre education.

Linda Hassall is Field of Study Coordinator Drama Major and Program Director Bachelor Creative Industries School HLSS Griffith University. She has 30 years of experience in the theatre industry as a director, playwright, and dramaturge. Linda's scholarly research lies in the relationship between scientific climate change themes and contemporary performance. A practice-led researcher, her artistic focus is on developing and analysing new work in Australian performance contexts from ecological and from ecocritical perspectives. Her research is also concerned with fostering sustainable production technologies in the theatre industry. She has recently published a book linking her artistic and scholarly practice: Theatres of Dust: Climate Gothic analysis in contemporary Australian drama and performance landscapes (2021). She is co-director of P+ERL, the Performance and Ecologies Research Lab, Griffith University, established with DRs Tanja Beer and Natalie Lazaroo.

Rand Hazou is a Palestinian theatre practitioner and scholar. His research explores arts engaging with rights and social justice. In 2004, Rand was commissioned by the UNDP to travel to the Occupied Territories in Palestine to work as a theatre consultant running workshops for Palestinian youths. In Aotearoa, he has led teaching and creative projects engaging with prison, aged-care, and street communities. Between 2019–2024, Rand was a researcher on the Health Research Council-funded research project 'Wellbeing and the Precariat', exploring the lived experiences of working families experiencing poverty and the impact this has on wellbeing. His current research explores the intersections between dignity and the arts. He is currently an Associate Professor at Massey University, Aotearoa, New Zealand.

Hobson Street Theatre Company is an award-winning theatre company created in partnership with the Auckland City Mission—Te Tāpui Atawhai, with an aim to tell stories that are full of manawa (heart), wairua (soul) and whakakata (humour). The HSTC was formed in 2010 from members of the street community accessing the homeless services, food assistance and health support provided by the Auckland City Mission. Central to the Company's vision is to use theatre to share the stories of the street community, and to foster dialogue on issues that lead to and perpetuate homelessness. Over the last twelve years, the Company has produced around ten productions and have received several awards. The company has toured to Wellington and Dunedin for successive Fringe Festival seasons and received awards including "Best Directed Chaos" (Wellington Fringe, 2018) and "Spirit of the Fringe" (Auckland, Fringe 2019). In 2019 the company was awarded the Arts Access Aotearoa Community Arts Award at the 2019 Te Putanga Toi Arts Access Awards. In 2023, they toured to the International Community Arts Festival in Rotterdam, where they worked in collaboration with Theater Pauluskerk.

Gillian Howell is a Senior Research Fellow in the Faculty of Fine Arts and Music, University of Melbourne, and a member of the Creativity and Wellbeing Research Initiative (CAWRI) Steering Committee. Her creative practice and applied research investigate how community music and other participatory arts can foster voice, dialogue, peacebuilding, and social repair in places impacted by war, disaster, and settler-colonialism.

She has worked as a research consultant and music leader around Australia and in many parts of the world including Bosnia-Herzegovina, Sri Lanka, Timor-Leste, Norway, Kosovo, and North Macedonia. Her publications appear in journals and books addressing community music, peace and conflict studies, music education, global development, and place-based community arts collaborations.

Michelle Johansson is a Tongan mother, theatre-maker, and educator. She serves as Kaitiaki at Ako Mātātupu: Teach First NZ, growing exceptional people to teach in low-decile schools. She is Kaiwhakahaere at Māia Centre for Social Justice and Education and the Creative Director of the Black Friars. South Auckland, decile-one born and bred, she is proud to work alongside amazing teachers, warriors, storytellers, and changemakers to re-story Pasifika in the largest Polynesian city in the world, to activate indigenous knowledges, to grow future leaders, and to hold courageous spaces for our young people to walk tall in all of their worlds.

Fran Kewene (Waikato-Maniapoto) identifies themselves as a creative Māori academic and locates their work in the intersections between hauora/health and whakaari Māori/theatre. Fran's work is wholistic and interdisciplinary using kaupapa Māori informed theatre methodologies and performance to examine equity, colonisation, and racism on the health and wellbeing of Māori and Indigenous peoples, and to privilege wairua (spirituality—connections) and non-spoken forms of communication. Fran is interested in the power-relationships inherent when evaluating community informed creative works operating on government or state funding.

Natalie Lazaroo is a Senior Lecturer in Drama and English Education at Griffith University. Her justice-oriented research work focuses on cultural and eco-citizenship, socially engaged performance, and decentring methodologies. Natalie is co-director of the Performance + Ecology Research Lab (P+ERL), which she established with her colleagues at the Creative Arts Research Institute (Griffith University). She is a member of the Creative Arts Research Institute and the Griffith Institute for Educational Research. Natalie is also a circus enthusiast and has performed in a number of circus shows with Vulcana Circus, including *Small Change* (2014) and *Circus in a Tea Cup* (2021, 2024).

Tony McCaffrey is a Lecturer at the National Academy of Singing and Dramatic Art, Ara Institute/Te Pukenga in Christchurch and, since 2004, director of Different Light Theatre. He is co-convenor of the Performance and Disability Working Group of the International Federation for Theatre Research. He is the author of Incapacity and Theatricality: Politics and Aesthetics in Theatre Involving Actors with Intellectual Disabilities (Routledge, 2019) and Giving and Taking Voice in Learning Disabled Theatre (Routledge, 2023).

Tristan Meecham is an artist who facilitates creative frameworks that enable social transformation; connecting community, audience, and artists together in events that transcend the everyday. He is the Director of All the Queens Men (with Bec Reid) that create spectacular theatrical and participatory arts experiences, championing social equality, celebrating diverse community through creative actions, and socially engaged frameworks.

Rebecca J. Moran is Lived Experience Engagement Fellow (NHMRC ALIVE) with the Big Anxiety Research Centre (BARC), University of New South Wales, Sydney. Bec has a long history as a mental health and justice reform advocate/activist, including utilising her lived experience of complex trauma to assist in teaching and training, with the aim of facilitating transformative learning experiences. Bec is passionate about co-design, collaboration, and the valuing of lived experience. Her PhD explores the ways people healing from trauma might find recognition and drive social change through social action and public testimony.

Jacqui Moyes (Tauiwi) is the Creative Director of Home Ground. With a background in community performing arts, prison arts programme coordination, and mentoring work with families engaged in social services, Jacqui co-created Home Ground in response to the social problems we face in Aotearoa New Zealand that are highlighted inside the justice system.

Molly Mullen is a Senior Lecturer at Waipapa Taumata Rau/University of Auckland. She has a professional background in children's theatre, youth theatre, applied theatre, and theatre and arts education. Much of her research now focuses on the intersection of policy, funding, and practice in applied theatre and other socially engaged art-making. She has published extensively on this topic, including a book, *Applied Theatre: Economies*, with Bloomsbury. She is co-editor of Research in Drama Education: The Journal of Applied Theatre and Performance.

Peta Murray is a late-blooming paracademic; Peta is a Lecturer and Researcher at RMIT University. She brings playwriting and theatre-making skills to bear in quest of new methods for communal conversation and collaborative practices. These approaches invite embodied experience, sensory immersion, and the witnessing afforded by live encounter. United under the concept of meaningful irreverence, her performable essays, secular rituals, and playful interventions create counternarratives for easing the way through major life transitions and navigating times of uncertainty.

Bec Reid (she/her) is third culture kid and an Australian-based Performer, Producer, Director, and Choreographer. Bec encourages people to experience their worlds in revelatory ways through highly physical, participatory, practical, and celebratory actions. For 20+ years, Bec has passionately collaborated where professional artists and communities coalesce, locally, nationally, and internationally. A WAAPA graduate, Bec began her professional career as Artistic Director of Stompin in Lutruwita (Tasmania), together with Luke George. Together with art wife Tristan Meecham, Bec is the co-Founder of All the Queens Men and with Ian Pidd and Kate McDonald, co-created Everybody NOW! Bec was Rimini Protokoll's Associate Director of reality-theatre juggernauts, 100% Melbourne (City of Melbourne), 100% Darwin (Darwin Festival), and 100% Brisbane (Museum of Brisbane) and has collaborated with Tracks Dance Company across 20+ years. Bec's true loves are Staffordshire Bull Terriers, Ceilidhs, and Italo Disco.

Kim Snider (she/they) is a doctoral candidate at Waipapa Taumata Rau University of Auckland. Kim's research focuses queer and critical arts-based research and uses drama and zine making methods to explore students' experiences of queer joy at school. In doing this work, she hopes to contribute to scholarship on the potential of creative methods in gender and sexuality research. Kim is also an experienced curriculum writer and mentor, and has facilitated workshops for educators in Australia, Austria, Canada, China, France, Japan, Aotearoa New Zealand, and the United Kingdom.

Elise Sterback is a PhD candidate at Waipapa Taumata Rau University of Auckland. Her research explores how embodied and creative processes, combined with a deeper understanding of living systems, can offer new ways to collectively envision the future and develop public policy. Elise previously ran an independent theatre venue in Auckland and has produced a range of theatre shows and art happenings. She is well known as a local arts advocate, currently serving on the board of regional arts trust Te Taumata Toi-a-iwi, and has participated in various arts policy steering groups at local and national levels.

Borni Te Rongopai Tukiwaho (Tūhoe, Te Arawa, Tuwharetoa) is an experienced producer, director, singer, and actor. He is educated in the arts and health sectors and has leadership roles in both industries with a national and international, published works to his credit. Borni works actively to help national organisations and artists build tools for self-sustainability resilience. He is currently working alongside, BATS Theatre, The Basement, Taki Rua, NZ Comedy Fest, Barbarian Productions, Te Taumata Toi-a-Iwi, and facilitates sustainability, conflict resolution, and hauora workshops in Auckland, Wellington, CHCH, and Dunedin. Borni is kaiwhakahaere for Taurima Vibes, is on the Health Promotion Agency National Māori Mental Health Advisory Panel, and is Director of the Auckland Fringe Festival.

Amber Walls is currently working as Youth Empowerment Advisor at Auckland Council, having completed an arts and youth wellbeing PhD at University of Auckland. Amber has spent most of her life working alongside young people who are marginalised to develop practices, policies, and cultures that enable them to thrive. Her PhD included working collaboratively with young people and arts, health, education, kaupapa Māori practitioners to co-design more culturally sustaining and mana-enhancing approaches to address youth mental health in Aotearoa. Amber is a founding member of Te Ora Auaha: Creative Wellbeing Alliance Aotearoa and Creative Collaborative, a platform for creatives to collaborate on social change initiatives.

Sarah Woodland is a Senior Lecturer in theatre at the Victorian College of the Arts, University of Melbourne, and a steering committee member of the Creativity and Wellbeing Research Initiative. Her research interests are applied theatre, socially engaged and participatory arts, with a particular focus on intercultural praxis towards justice and wellbeing. Sarah teaches undergraduate and postgraduate theatre courses and has published extensively in the fields of applied theatre and participatory arts. She is co-editor of the journal *Australasian Drama Studies.*

List of Figures

Fig. 2.1	An image of Mary Miller from the film *Two Minutes of Ordinary Everyday Life*. Image by Paul McCaffrey (2024)	32
Fig. 2.2	An image of Angie sitting with her Māori birth mother. Image by Angelia Douglas (n.d.)	46
Fig. 3.1	*Southside Rise* poster, by L. Folau and F. Fifita (2017). Reprinted with permission	52
Fig. 4.1	The coming back out salon by All The Queens Men for Sydney World Pride. Image by Bryony Jackson (2023)	74
Fig. 4.2	LGBTIQ+ Elders dance club by All The Queens Men, Melbourne. Image by Bryony Jackson (2019)	81
Fig. 4.3	The Coming Back Out Ball by All The Queens Men, Melbourne Town Hall. Image by Bryony Jackson (2018)	87
Fig. 5.1	Hearts on display. Artwork created by women who have participated in a variety of Home Ground projects. Photo credit: Rebecca McMillan (2024)	98
Fig. 5.2	Home Ground evaluation lei. Photo credit: Rebecca McMillan (2024)	108
Fig. 7.1	Community Economy Return on investment (Gibson-Graham et al., 2013)	142
Fig. 7.2	Simplified mauri ora assessment tool. From Dombroski et al. (2022, p. 14)	145
Fig. 7.3	Exhibition montage	146

Fig. 8.1 Te Whare Tapa Whā or The House of Four Sides—a holistic model of Māori Health developed by Sir Mason Durie based on the metaphor of the wharenui or meeting house. Image credit: Jeanne Leclercq (2021) 163
Fig. 9.1 Visual representation of project X ToC. Image credit: Amber Walls (2021) 183
Fig. 9.2 Mana Taiohi Auaha: A creative youth wellbeing practice framework for Aotearoa. Designed by: Asha Munn (2023) 188
Fig. 10.1 Socio-ecological model [SEM] for "voice" in the lives of adolescents affected by conflict in Lebanon, Jordan, and Türkiye. Developed by G. Howell, based on Bronfenbrenner (1977) 200
Fig. 10.2 Descriptive and metaphoric labels chosen at a workshop in Jordan. Image by A. Mokdad 203
Fig. 10.3 Girls aged 14–17 years in Za'atari Camp record their song. Image by A. Mokdad 206
Fig. 11.1 "From Elsewhere." Dr. Natalie Lazaroo and Sophie Whitecross are tumbled by sling artist Chloë Callistemon to represent the washing up of debris on the shores of Moreton Bay. Image by Dr. Kaya Barry (2023) 227
Fig. 11.2 Site visit to Pinkenba. Artist Researcher Dr. Natalie Lazaroo is searching for evidence of where the Curlew has landed. Image by Dr. Kaya Barry (2023) 234

List of Tables

Table 8.1 The Hobson Street Theatre company evaluation framework 165

Table 8.2 Prompts that can be used in a continuum exercise where participants are asked to place themselves on an imaginary scale and where one side of the room designates 'strongly agree' and the opposing side 'strongly disagree' 168

CHAPTER 1

Introduction: Re-evaluating Evaluation

Molly Mullen, Sarah Woodland, and Rand Hazou

In September 2023, the editors of this volume convened the 'Precarity, Creative Arts, and Wellbeing Symposium' at Massey University in Auckland. The two-day hui (gathering) brought together scholars and arts practitioners mainly from Aotearoa New Zealand (Aotearoa NZ) and Australia to share approaches to working in precarious settings as well as innovative methods for researching and evaluating the impact of participatory arts[1] on the wellbeing of precarious communities. The symposium

[1] We acknowledge that 'participatory arts' is broad term that can often be associated with performance that engages audiences as participants. In this book, we draw on Francois Matarasso's useful definition of participatory arts simply as the creation of an artwork by professional artists and non-professional artists (2019, 48).

M. Mullen (✉)
University of Auckland, Auckland, New Zealand
e-mail: m.mullen@auckland.ac.nz

S. Woodland
University of Melbourne, Melbourne, VIC, Australia
e-mail: sarah.woodland@unimelb.edu.au

R. Hazou
Massey University, Auckland, New Zealand
e-mail: R.T.Hazou@massey.ac.nz

M. Mullen et al. (eds.), *Artful Evaluation for Creative Health and Wellbeing*, New Directions in Cultural Policy Research,
https://doi.org/10.1007/978-3-032-17063-7_1

was the culmination of a series of attempts to bring together the wider discourse about the role and value of the arts, and concerns with what seemed to be increasing precarity and instability in the social and cultural contexts of both Aotearoa NZ and Australia. It felt important to us that rethinking the role and value of the arts in relation to these contextual changes would involve rethinking why and how the arts were evaluated. Little did we know that this would lead to us producing this book.

Our symposium was, of course, part of a bigger picture. It aimed to contribute in creative and scholarly ways to ongoing arts, health, and wellbeing work in Aotearoa NZ and Australia. This includes the advocacy, research, and other sector-level action being led by the likes of Te Ora Auaha: Creative Wellbeing Alliance Aotearoa, the Arts and Wellbeing Research and Evaluation Network (Aotearoa NZ and Australia), Arts Access Aotearoa, VicHealth (Australia), and Creative Australia. It also includes the work of individual organisations, artists, and practitioners who keep developing, discussing, and sharing ways of working, because they can sense what they are doing is making a difference. And there are researchers, often working alongside, through or in partnership with creative practice. Together, this work has succeeded in raising the prominence of the relationship between the arts, health, and wellbeing broadly, as well as developing and promoting locally distinct practice approaches and frameworks.

What do we see, then, as the distinguishing features or strengths of arts, health, and wellbeing work in Australia and Aotearoa NZ, which have informed our decision to focus this book on this part of the world? First, there is the dynamic, strong tradition of **Indigenous-led research and practice**, as well as the examples of, and frameworks for, equitable, generative **Indigenous–non-Indigenous collaboration**. Another notable feature is the prevalence of successful **cross-disciplinary and cross-sector solidarity**, and examples of initiatives that have led to meaningful connections and conversations between what can be deeply divided domains: research, policy, and practice. And, finally, we suggest, it is now the norm, rather than the exception, to understand **health and wellbeing as holistic and as contingent on equity and justice**.

These features were clear at the 'Precarity, Creative Arts, and Wellbeing Symposium'. For example, Fran Kewene gave a keynote presenting her kaupapa Māori theatre research praxis. Grounded in Māori hauora frameworks and drawing on both Māori and Western theatre traditions, Kewene challenges health inequities and promotes changes within health and social care to better foster Māori vitality. Hobson Street Theatre Company's verbatim drama, *Un-Welfare State*, performed at the conference, presented research drawn from the three-year research project 'Wellbeing and the Precariat', which was funded by the Health Research Council of New Zealand. The interdisciplinary research team included seven principal researchers and eight postgraduate students from three Aotearoa New Zealand universities. These researchers, from Psychology, Kaupapa Māori, and Theatre backgrounds, interviewed low-income households about their experiences of health and wellbeing. These interviews became the basis of a verbatim drama exploring experiences of the welfare system in Aotearoa NZ and highlighting the apparent deficit of care within an increasingly punitive welfare system. Dr Ying Wang, meanwhile, shared how her work to support the wellbeing of Asian communities in Aotearoa NZ involves working across the arts, health, and creative arts therapies, drawing from Eastern and Western philosophies and therapeutic practices. All these examples share a focus on equity and a **prominent concern with collective or community wellbeing**, which we identify as another feature of the arts, health, and wellbeing ecosystem in Australia and Aotearoa NZ.

Another keynote presentation at the symposium was given by Adrian Jackson, founder and former director of Cardboard Citizens, a UK-based Theatre Company that produces work particularly by, with, and for those who have experienced homelessness, inequity, or poverty. A specialist in the Theatre of the Oppressed, Jackson has translated five books by the Brazilian theatre pioneer Augusto Boal and specialises in the use of participatory arts as an inclusive practice to engage marginalised communities. As part of his keynote, Jackson shared an anecdote about the Peckham Experiment. Led by two doctors, George Scott Williamson and Innes Pearse—who established the Pioneer Health Centre in Peckham, London, in the 1930s—the Peckham Experiment involved the study of factors that promoted and enhanced health. As part of his keynote, Jackson shared an anecdote about how the doctors leading the Peckham Experiment were interested in measuring 'the spring in a person's step' or the 'gleam in a person's eye', as potential indicators that people are living healthy lives.

The Pioneer Health Centre was closed in 1950 and much of the data on the Peckham Experiment was lost in the Second World War (Feedland 2007). This might explain the difficulty in trying to verify the anecdote shared by Jackson. Despite our inability to confirm the provenance of this story, the account is nevertheless intriguing. It is a story that conveys what seems to be an ongoing challenge for Western health practices, to recognise and 'account for' the more elusive qualities and conditions that comprise health and wellbeing, to give them greater value. The story resonated with many attendees of the symposium. It pointed to the often intangible but still observable, or otherwise discernible, value that participating in the arts can have for those involved. Ask any artist, arts educator, facilitator, or community participant who has been moved by an art project to describe its 'effect', and they may well resort to adjectives with bodily and affective dimensions. For example, they might report that the atmosphere of the art project has become lighter, that they felt a 'quickening of the spirit' or became 'more alive'. An artist running an arts project might notice a sense of pride emerging, registered in a shift in comportment, heads held higher, or a new willingness to make eye contact. Participants may feel more attuned to each other, their bodies more 'open' or relaxed, a renewed willingness and capacity to listen. Adrian Jackson's story made us reflect on how such things often remain elusive to standard evaluation methods; things which we, as artists, arts educators, and participants, think/feel/know are important in arts practice.

In keeping with the features and strengths of our regional context, this book presents practice-based and practice-led[2] research from Aotearoa NZ and Australia, which critically explores the contribution that participation in the arts makes to wellbeing and health. By 'critically', we mean research that explicitly addresses the social, political, cultural and economic factors that underlie (a) people's ill health and poor wellbeing, (b) the kinds of practices, methodologies, and knowledge that are privileged, and (c) issues of power and positionality. By 'participation in the arts' we mean the active involvement of people in a creative process. We acknowledge that other forms of participation in the arts (e.g. as an audience member) also contribute to health and wellbeing. But, perhaps because of our common background in applied theatre,[3] we are particularly interested in the value of people taking part in creative arts processes

[2] Here we distinguish between practice-based research which prioritises research as coming out of the practice, whereas practice-led research prioritises the practice as the main mode of inquiry (See Nelson 2013).

[3] Applied Theatre is theatre that usually happens outside of conventional theatre spaces, in social and community contexts, with diverse groups of people, in order to bring about social change.

that have a meaningful connection to their everyday lives and experiences. This book also presents ideas, examples, and models for evaluating the contribution of the arts to health and wellbeing in ways that take experiential, embodied, and artistic ways of knowing seriously, as well as methods of evaluation that are sensitive and relevant to the complex cultural, creative, and ecological contexts within which practice unfolds.

The Shifting Landscape of Arts, Health, and Wellbeing

Of course, the conversations and concerns that emerged at the 'Precarity, Creative Arts, and Wellbeing Symposium' happened in dialogue with the wider issues and debates unfolding in Australia, Aotearoa NZ, and internationally at that time. It's not possible to give a comprehensive overview of this sometimes drastically shifting landscape of policy, practice, and research, but we think it is useful to highlight some key points.

In Aotearoa NZ, a policy 'turn to wellbeing' was prompted by the sixth Aotearoa New Zealand Labour government, who, under the leadership of Prime Minister Jacinda Adern, launched the world's first Wellbeing Budget in 2019, making Aotearoa NZ the first country to measure success by its people's wellbeing (Roy 2019). The Wellbeing Budget signalled a shift to a more holistic consideration of the factors that contribute to citizens living good lives. It also marked a shift in how the government would measure policy and funding outcomes and their contribution to Aotearoa NZ's living standards.[4] Jacinda Ardern also took on the ministerial portfolio for Arts, Culture and Heritage, and her early speeches in this role emphasised the importance of the arts to public wellbeing, people's sense of identity, and social change (Ardern 2018). Her statements generated more interest in and recognition of the relationship between arts and wellbeing. They did not, however, lead to the re-conceptualisation of the role and value of the arts or, importantly, how they should be funded.

The COVID-19 pandemic disrupted the further embedding of wellbeing as the Ardern government's policy driver. The pandemic and its global reverberations also contributed to a sense of increased urgency in

[4] "The LSF is a flexible framework that prompts our thinking about policy impacts across the different dimensions of wellbeing, as well as the long-term and distributional issues and implications of policy". https://www.treasury.govt.nz/information-and-services/nz-economy/higher-living-standards/our-living-standards-framework.

Aotearoa NZ, Australia, and internationally to consider the importance of the arts to the health of communities as well as the precarious situation of arts workers within our societies. Some of the initiatives that were put in place to support artists and arts organisations through the pandemic and in its immediate aftermath indicated that change was possible. For example, a new three-year fund in Aotearoa NZ for organisations providing access to the arts for marginalised communities enabled both growth and sustainability.[5] In Australia, the conservative government provided 200 million AUD in support through the 'RISE' Fund, but this was criticised by many for its focus on large commercial entertainment companies over independent artists and small-to-medium organisations. Meanwhile, more and more evidence stacked up showing multiple health, wellbeing, economic (and more) benefits from participating in the arts, and increasingly how such benefits were achieved (Arts Access Aotearoa 2024; Carter et al. 2024; Creative Australia 2023; Creative New Zealand 2023). But, as any temporary COVID-19-related boosts to funding and support for the arts and artists came to an end, the situation seemed just as, if not more, precarious than before the pandemic (Morrow 2022; Mullen and Lythberg 2021). And, beyond the arts, the post-pandemic years have brought recessions, political polarisation, climate change impacts, and international conflicts. Across many countries, social and individual stability and other important pre-conditions—or determinants—of health and wellbeing seem to be in decline (World Health Organisation 2025).

In the face of these crises, there have been moves towards strengthening 'arts and health' as a field, and a significant area of policy and practice. In Australia, arts and health began to emerge through community arts and health promotion work through the 1970s and 1980s, followed by hospital arts programmes in the 1990s. The field then started to gain prominence through the work of Margaret Meagher, who established Arts and Health Australia, and the first international conference in 2009. Since then, policy attention has grown, with the establishment in 2014 of the National Arts and Health Framework[6]; state-level leadership from bodies like VicHealth; and Creative Australia's *Creating*

[5] https://artsaccess.org.nz/Investment-in-creative-spaces-pays-dividends-in-health-and-social-outcomes.

[6] https://www.arts.qld.gov.au/images/documents/artsqld/Research/National-Arts-and-Health-Framework-May-2014.pdf.

Wellbeing report (Creative Australia 2023), which identifies the challenges and opportunities of arts approaches to wellbeing and informs their 2024 request for tender supporting the development of creative health practice.[7] There has also been a growth in state-wide arts and health networks to connect practitioners and scholars across the sector. While the Australian Government's most recent cultural policy, *Revive*, does not promote a standalone arts and health programme, it encourages cross-sector collaboration and integration of the arts into various social settings, including healthcare (Australian Government 2023). At the time of writing, Creative Australia announced a two-year arts and health initiative whose goal is to 'strengthen the role of the arts in health and community care' (Creative Australia 2025). These initiatives have been informed by advances in university-level arts and health education, research and leadership, including through organisations like the Big Anxiety Research Centre (University of New South Wales) and the Creativity and Wellbeing Research Initiative (University of Melbourne). Some universities are driving an interest in social prescribing (Forbes et al. 2025) and public health initiatives that promote the arts (see, for example, Good Arts Good Mental Health in Western Australia).[8] In Australia, these recent developments are being driven by a renewed sense of urgency post-pandemic, including a national mental health crisis and the rapidly escalating wellbeing impacts brought about by climate change. In Aotearoa NZ, the field remains less explicitly defined, being characterised more by informal alliances and networks (like Te Ora Auaha: Creative Wellbeing Alliance), sustained advocacy and practice innovation,[9] but a lack of direct policy on arts and health or wellbeing (Walls 2023).

Rather than radical shifts in the scholarly discourse of arts, health, and wellbeing, what we want to highlight are perhaps better described as

[7] https://creative.gov.au/sites/creative-Australia/files/documents/2025-05/Supporting%20Creative%20Health%20Practice%20in%20Australia%20-%20Request%20for%20Tender.pdf.

[8] https://goodartsgoodmentalhealth.com.au/.

[9] See, for example, Creative Waikato Standing Up for the Arts https://creativewaikato.co.nz/advocacy/standing-up-for-the-arts, and Creative NZ: Arts Council New Zealand Toi Aotearoa advocacy campaigns https://creativenz.govt.nz/advocating-for-the-arts/our-advocacy-work.

growing trends. One trend we observe is towards increasing critical scholarship. Acknowledging that critical perspectives have been an important and continuous feature of arts and health scholarship (Parr 2017), there seems to be growing recognition that when the discourse on arts, health, and wellbeing centres uncritically on decontextualised individual or environmental factors, structural determinants and systemic failings can be ignored. This recognition is perhaps leading to more research addressing whether and how the arts contribute to health equity (Sunderland et al. 2018) and community or ecological wellbeing (Gattenhof et al. 2021). Indigenous research and practice are also increasingly prominent (Van Styvendale et al. 2021; Bartleet, Sunderland and Lakhani 2018), as is research highlighting the cultural specificity of conceptions of health and wellbeing, and decolonial approaches, which we explore in more detail below. Taken together, these trends present a substantial move to challenge and displace some of the paradigms and conceptions of value that have dominated the field, a movement this book seeks to contribute to.

Rethinking how Value is Theorised, Measured, and Communicated

This book engages with international conversations about cultural value, which call into question traditional approaches and assumptions about what the arts are and why they matter (Belfiore 2020; Crossick and Kaszynska 2016; Meyrick et al. 2018). This book, then, is not an evaluation toolkit. Instead, it presents examples and case studies where evaluating arts participation has involved interrogating notions of value. This is, we argue, an important step towards aligning what is *of value* to the participants and artists involved in arts, health, and wellbeing practices, with the methods used to evaluate those practices. It is about putting the values back in evaluation. Some research and evaluation approaches, largely in the positivist tradition, claim to produce value-neutral findings (House and Howe 1999). Research in the positivist tradition requires the researcher to be objective, to ensure their values do not influence the study in any way. Feminist, Queer, Indigenous, and other critical scholarship has responded to these claims by showing that all methodologies and methods used in research and evaluation are shaped by values (Bhavnani 1993; Smith 2012). Nicola Bright and Sally Boyd (2024) explain this problem as a feature of the health sector more broadly, where "Western approaches often appear to position measurement tools as 'culture free' and appropriate for everyone, when, in reality, they are founded on the culture and values of a dominant culture" (p. 4). Feminist science scholars, meanwhile, show how the 'instruments' used in research (from equipment used for science experiments to research questionnaires) are not neutral tools for measuring something. Rather, they are complex social *and* material practices that play a part in producing what is 'found' or not (Bhavnani 1993). James Vincent (2022) makes a similar point in his social history of measurement, suggesting that "measurement is a mirror to society itself; it is a form of attention that reveals what we value in the world" (5). In this book, then, scholars, artists, and allied practitioners are asking what counts, and what is not counted by the tools and frameworks that we work with.

It seems important to end this section with a caveat. While we think anyone involved in evaluating the contributions participatory arts might make to health and wellbeing must think carefully and critically before adopting some of the dominant approaches, we are in no way calling for the outright rejection of methodologies premised on objectivity or of quantitative methods. Instead, we draw attention to examples where scholars, artists, and other practitioners are rethinking these concepts. For example, Indigenous scholars are developing Indigenous and decolonial quantitative methods,[10] and feminist scholars reconceive objectivity as situated knowledges (Bhavnani 1993). Collaborative, transdisciplinary research in the US has resulted in 'Data Theatre', using theatre as a means for communities to 'translate' quantitative research data, sparking reflection and debate and informing public policy (Snyder-Young et al. 2024). Our concern, outlined further below, is that particular sets of values, or conceptions of value, can become so ubiquitous in evaluation that they are left unscrutinised. This, then, delimits our priorities when working with communities through artistic practice, while appearing to serve our practice by generating evidence.

What Counts? The Impact of Impact Evaluation

We are as susceptible as anyone to believing that if we can produce enough of the right kind of evidence through our research, we can inform policy change, or other kinds of change, in a way that will lead to better

[10] For example, the Civic Laboratory, https://civiclaboratory.nl/methodological-projects/indigenous-quantitive-methods/#project-background.

outcomes for communities and perhaps better support and resourcing for the arts. The fact that government agencies sometimes even commission this research makes us feel like, if we just get it right, it could really make a difference. But, as we outline above, even though the evidence piles up, policy changes based on that evidence feel as far off as ever.

Writing about the UK, Eleonora Belfiore (2022, 294) puts our experience into the context of the evidence-based policy trend, which originated in the 1990s in health, and has subsequently 'gone global':

> Despite the move towards a supposedly "evidence-based" policy, "evidence" rarely underpins decision-making, especially in policies surrounding the perceived social impacts of the arts. Rather than enhancing accountability and transparency in policy making, the pressures placed on English publicly funded cultural institutions to produce evaluations of their performance, and to subject themselves to the constant attempt to measure their efficiency and impact, has been pivotal in the escalation of very dubious 'evidence'. (Belfiore 2022, 294)

Belfiore argues that evidence-based policymaking privileges objective, standardised, quantified, linear ways of knowing over the rich, subjective, experiential ways of knowing that come from the arts and humanities and, we would add, from an Australian and Aotearoa NZ perspective, over Indigenous ways of knowing. The image depicted in the above quote is familiar to us, of the immense pressure experienced by arts and cultural organisations to prove their worth, to justify their receiving public or philanthropic funds, by providing evidence of their impact. Indeed, in Aotearoa NZ and Australia, understandings of the value of *participatory arts*, of arts that bring together social and artistic aims and processes, have been almost completely captured by the social impact paradigm. It is almost impossible to articulate the way the arts might lead to change, make a difference, in any other way.

The social impact paradigm emerged in the 1990s as public policymaking became tied to the imperative for governments to demonstrate that their policies were delivering value for money (Patton 2023). Applied to the arts, the social impact paradigm creates the requirement "to deliver economic or other public benefits…in return for societal support through dedicated institutions and funding" (Belfiore 2015, 95–6). Beyond government, philanthropists and charitable trusts now describe their giving as a form of social impact investment, requiring measurable evidence of social returns (impacts). Taken at face value, of course, governments and charities need to be held accountable for how they spend people's taxes or donations, and, of course, this means they have to require anyone using those funds to provide evidence that the money has been well spent. And, perhaps it is a good way to get institutions that can be perceived to be too insular or elitist, like academia and the arts, to be more concerned about being of use to society. However, as Gedutis et al. (2023) argue, the social impact paradigm is less concerned with ensuring that research benefits society, and "more a specific form of evaluation linked to an economic theory of society based on accountability and a mechanistic a-political (or anti-democratic) evaluation" (32). Gedutis et al. describe social impact evaluation as anti-democratic because decisions about what is of value and how it will be judged are rarely subject to public discussion; rarely are they determined either by the people running an art or research project, let alone the people such projects are intended to benefit.

Our hope is that producing this book might help displace the social impact paradigm as the dominant way of understanding value, and, in doing so, contribute to widening the space of possibility for evaluating participatory arts. Debates about what counts as evidence and what evidence counts have been ongoing in the field and literature of arts and health. For example, Anni Raw et al. (2012) propose that the somewhat obsessive, narrow focus on generating quantitative evidence of the impact of arts on health and wellbeing has detracted from the much-needed theorisation of that practice. Meanwhile, leading arts and health scholars Stephen Clift et al. (2021) argue that concerns about the conceptualisation of impact in arts and health research and evaluation, which were raised as early as the 1990s, have still not been addressed in the 2020s. They highlight, for example, the "danger in the arts and health literature of 'psychologising' social and health issues and failing to see the larger public health picture with the central role played by underlying economic and social structural causes of inequalities" (454). They also note the ways in which issues of "aesthetics and quality of arts engagement" are given no attention in key reports that claim to present evidence for the health impacts of the arts (454). What we take from these debates is a call for a richer range of methodologies, and for theorisation and forms of evidence that will genuinely deepen and enrich the knowledge and practice of our field.

Beyond Impact: Emerging Methodologies

As discussed above, the social impact paradigm's dominance, along with the pressing demands of neoliberal funding and accountability structures, has led to prioritising the instrumental over intrinsic value of the arts in health and social sectors. This has often led to a reliance on evaluation measures that reduce the rich and complex experience of participating in the arts to a digestible package of positively spun statistics, impact stories, images, and soundbites. While this kind of evaluation in arts and health/wellbeing seems to persist, several trends in academic or scholarly research have informed a shift in how we might approach the ethical, aesthetic, and economic values underpinning such practices; and the ways in which we might conceive, measure, and articulate value (evaluate). We briefly outline these trends below, focusing on the development and legitimisation of **artistic practice in scholarly research**; a proliferation of **practice-led participant-centred or participant-led methods** in health and social research; a growing call for **transdisciplinary knowledge creation** in addressing complex real-world problems; and the rise of **Indigenous knowledges** and culturally grounded methodologies to address the needs of First Nations communities.

Artistic Practice in Scholarly Research

Concurrently with the emergence of the social impact paradigm in the arts sectors in the 1990s—at least in Western universities—there also emerged a movement towards the arts in qualitative research. Arts-informed research (Cole and Knowles 2008), arts-based research (ABR) (Leavy 2020), and arts-based health research (ABHR) (Boydell et al. 2016) incorporate artistic practices and creative processes into research methodologies. These approaches highlight the affective, sensory, and embodied aspects of data collection and analysis. Creative practice as research (or practice-led research) also developed in the academy as the arts disciplines rapidly expanded in higher education and scholars sought to legitimise creative practice as a rigorous form of inquiry (Nelson 2013). This centring of artistic or arts-led research methods in the generation of knowledge was applied to the development of artistic practices and disciplines themselves, as well as to the wider social, political, and philosophical questions underpinning our experiences of the world. Consequently, there has been a proliferation of creative and artistic research methods such as autoethnography (Ellis et al. 2011), photovoice (Catalani and Minkler 2010), digital storytelling (Hardy and Sumner 2017), poetic inquiry (Prendergast et al. 2009), ethnodrama or ethnotheatre (Saldaña 2011), research-based theatre (Beck et al. 2011), and applied theatre as research (Anderson and O'Connor 2014). These methods centre the creative exploration of one's own and others' lived experiences through different artistic disciplines. While the social impact paradigm may have led to a narrowing of what counts, the flourishing of creative arts in research has broadened considerations of what is of value and how we might capture it.

Practice-Led and Participant-Led Methods

A rise in practice-based qualitative methods, such as action research in education, health, and social care settings, placed an emphasis on evaluating existing practices with a view to improving and refining them. As these applied research approaches developed, concern for redressing the power imbalances inherent in the researcher/researched or 'professional'/'client' relationship began to emerge, resulting in participatory qualitative research methods such as participatory action research (PAR), which seeks to centre the lived experiences of professionals and end-users in evaluating the efficacy of programmes (Kemmis and McTaggart 2005). Similarly, 'developmental evaluation', as conceptualised by Michael Quinn Patton (2011), offers a flexible and adaptive approach to evaluating complex, innovative initiatives in dynamic environments. This approach emphasises real-time feedback, learning, and adaptation, evolving in response to participants' needs and emerging insights (Gamble 2008). Such participatory methods are flexible and responsive, empowering traditionally marginalised voices (nurses, patients, teachers, students, and more) with the authority to contribute new knowledge that will influence policy and practice. This, in turn, has evolved into the co-design movement in research and public policy, where (at its best) the beneficiaries and stakeholders in health and social care work alongside researchers, practitioners, and policymakers to develop programmes; establish shared articulations of value/s and success indicators for those programmes; collaborate in developing methods for evaluating programme efficacy in meeting those indicators; and work together to interpret the findings (Zamenopoulos and Alexiou 2018). Nevertheless, 'co-design' has replaced 'community consultation' as a buzz word in health and social programme development, sometimes leading to tokenistic efforts to engage participants in such processes. Our book foregrounds ethical participant-centred evaluative practices that promote genuine collaboration and co-design, with a recognition that such approaches involve nurturing meaningful and trusting relationships over time.

Transdisciplinary Knowledges

In applied theatre, we have seen a consistent theme of collaboration across disciplines in practice-led explorations of how the arts might enhance professional practice in health, education, and other sectors; or how they might serve to articulate the lived experiences, needs, and priorities of stakeholders. Collaborations between theatre makers/scholars and, for example, scholars and practitioners in social work, nursing, medicine, environmental sciences, and many more emphasise the power of the arts in accessing embodied modes of learning and knowing that reach beyond traditional didactic pedagogies ('chalk and talk') or research methods such as surveys, interviews, and focus groups (Prendergast et al. 2024). And emerging art/science collaborations are giving rise to innovative technologies and transdisciplinary knowledges that push beyond the scope of what one discipline might achieve alone in understanding, for example, the potential uses of virtual reality in healing Indigenous intergenerational trauma (Menezes 2024), or the use of sound in measuring the impacts of climate change on communities and ecosystems (Barclay 2019). In response to increasingly complex social relations and geopolitical upheavals, we recognise the need to continue working collaboratively, co-creating knowledges and innovations across disciplines.

Indigenous Knowledges

A growing body of research supports the effectiveness of community-driven, arts-based programmes in health and wellbeing promotion and education among First Nations communities in Australia and Aotearoa NZ, particularly in response to existing health inequities (Carr et al. 2025; Durie 2004; Hickey et al. 2021; McEwan et al. 2013; Sunderland et al. 2023; Verbunt et al. 2021; Woodland and Bell-Wykes 2024). These approaches recognise the unique strengths and perspectives of First

Nations communities in addressing their own health challenges. Indigenous frameworks, such as centring Country and relational accountability, challenge the ontological hegemony of Western science (Harriden 2023). By prioritising relationality and reciprocity, these frameworks offer a more holistic understanding of wellbeing, the natural world, and the interconnectedness of human and more-than-human experiences. With an emphasis on cultural determinants of health (Sunderland et al. 2023), much of this work has embraced and adapted arts-led and participatory methods such as poetic enquiry (Cooms and Saunders 2024), 'Aboriginal participatory action research' (APAR) (Dudgeon et al. 2020), developmental evaluation (McKegg et al. 2016), and applied theatre as research (Woodland et al. 2024). While not the sole focus of this volume, we acknowledge the growing calls for programme evaluations in First Nations communities to engage with Indigenous methodologies that respect and honour these culturally grounded knowledge systems; and we draw inspiration from the collaborations we have undertaken with our First Nations colleagues and mentors in this space.

We argue that the trends described above have inspired and informed the arts-led evaluative practices discussed in this book, providing a roadmap for how we and others have arrived at the idea of 'artful evaluation'.

Arriving at 'Artful Evaluation'

We have called this book *Artful Evaluation*, embracing the multiple connotations of the word artful: to be creative, skilful, and wise, but also crafty and strategic. It encompasses critical and creative approaches to framing, exploring, uncovering, and articulating the 'measures' or indicators of value in creative wellbeing projects. Artful evaluation implies a certain agility in working with communities and participants, enabling the evaluation process itself to enhance wellbeing through genuine collaborative processes that are inclusive and empowering. It also involves artfully integrating evaluation processes with art-making, collapsing traditional distinctions between process and outcome, art-making and meaning-making, or knowledge creation and knowledge sharing. It may also imply the nuanced skill, articulated in some of this book's chapters, of evaluating in ways that serve both the extrinsic requirements of funders and the goals and values determined by the artists and participants.

An emphasis on the 'art' in artful evaluation moves us towards considering the aesthetic, affective, embodied, and imaginative qualities inherent in artistic practices. These qualities can enhance evaluation processes to generate deeper, more nuanced accounts of complex experiences. Many of the contributions to this volume emphasise holism in conceiving artful evaluation, resisting the reductive tendency to categorise or silo that is present in much traditional evaluation. This holistic approach reflects the formal quality of an artwork that often generates an integrated whole while conveying a variety of different meanings to different audiences. We now turn to the contributions to this volume, highlighting how they advance this idea of 'artful evaluation' through a range of practices and approaches.

Chapter Summaries

Section 1: What is of Value?

The two chapters in this section ask challenging questions about the value systems that are built into policy, funding, and evaluation. The first chapter is a personal account written by **Tony McCaffrey,** exploring the work Different Light Theatre, a mixed ability theatre company based in Ōtautahi Christchurch, Aotearoa NZ. The chapter considers the 'value' of disabled theatre and explores the tension between the difficulties of physical and cognitive impairment, and the benefits afforded to disabled people in theatrical performance. McCaffrey questions the evaluation of the aesthetic and political efficacy of disability performance according to mechanistic models of input and output and of profit and loss. In contrast, he notes the importance of the gift economy, which sustains the labour of Different Light Theatre and the bonds of love, obligation, commitment, and mutual care that continue to inform their work.

Tongan mother, educator, and theatre maker, **Michelle Johansson**, meticulously unpacks the policy and funding context in Aotearoa NZ, exposing just how and why it continues to fail Pacific artists and young people in South Auckland. This chapter shows how even progressive policies that pertain to Pacific Peoples and Pacific arts perpetuate colonial value systems. With reference to Johansson's work with the Black Friars theatre company, and the Southside Rise project, this chapter challenges policymakers to take up Indigenous concepts, methods, and scholarship if they really want to recognise and value the strengths and knowledge of Pacific Peoples and their arts.

Section 2: Justice-Oriented Evaluation

The next three chapters all present examples of deeply critical and equity orientated approaches to evaluation. The contribution from **Peta Murray, Marnie Badham, Tristan Meecham, and Bec Reid** proposes a 'queevaluation' framework for understanding the value and significance of socially engaged arts projects like those created by the Australian company, All The Queens Men. Rather than imposing narrow impact measurement approaches, queevaluation embraces queer theory, participatory methodologies, and creative practices grounded in ethics, care, and self-determination. Their approach illuminates unexpected dimensions like enhanced social connection, intergenerational knowledge sharing, identity affirmation, and revealed advocacy needs.

Jacqui Moyes and Fran Kewene's chapter offers a critical but heartfelt reflection on the evaluative practices developed by Home Ground, who run arts-informed programmes with wāhine (women) in Aotearoa NZ's criminal justice system. They describe their evaluation as happening in the liminal, transitional spaces between prison and community, and as always trying to balance imperatives from their practice, from the lived experiences of all involved, and from funders. The creative approach to evaluation developed by Home Ground is orientated towards clearly articulated values and guiding principles, and an understanding of the contribution made by participatory arts to health and wellbeing that is firmly located in the context of Te Tiriti o Waitangi (the founding settlement document of Aotearoa NZ).

Poppy de Souza and Bec Moran propose a justice-oriented framework for valuing lived experience expertise and co-creative practices attuned to the politics of voice within the evidence of experience in health and wellbeing. The chapter focuses on the authors' respective projects: de Souza's Holding Breath, which used voice-note exchanges co-created with Long COVID-19 patients, and Moran's video installation Big Grief, Big Horror about experiencing family trauma. Through these two case studies, the chapter positions listening, witnessing, and creative repair as central principles. They prioritise the value of 'slow attention, mutual witnessing, and creative reparation' in the wake of structural harm, stigma, and grief to propose 'creative reparation' through practices that do not reproduce harm and hold transformative potential.

Section 3: Community Wellbeing, Participation and Self-Determination

This section shares four examples of evaluative processes where conceptions of wellbeing and frameworks for evaluation have been developed through participatory and collaborative processes.

Kelly Dombroski reflects on her experience developing and applying an approach to evaluating the work of a non-governmental, place-making, and arts-enabling organisation, Life in Vacant Spaces. This chapter provides an example of how the notions of 'investments' and 'returns' might be taken back from the impact paradigm and repurposed so as to account holistically for the value that creative initiatives bring to community wellbeing.

The chapter by **Rand Hazou and members of the Hobson Street Theatre Company** (HSTC) details how the company developed their own evaluation model focusing on aspects of wellbeing which will help them evaluate the success of workshops, rehearsals, and creative projects over time. A key feature of HSTC's work is its engagement with the 'street' and with the community accessing services from the Auckland City Mission. As such, they are often facilitating theatre workshops and projects with a community impacted by multiple forms of precarity and health impacts. The chapter details how these considerations not only impact on the company's ability to evaluate aspects of its work as well as how 'data' is collected, but also how a focus on wellbeing informed the development of their evaluation model.

The chapter by **Amber Walls** and **Borni Te Rongopai Tukiwaho** shares insights about an evaluation framework that was developed for Project X—a creative programme for young people experiencing mental health challenges in Aotearoa NZ. The framework unpacks the participatory research methods used to develop a framework for evaluating Project X, which could articulate 'impacts' in ways that were evidence-informed, aligned with participants' aspirations, and reflective of the unique contribution of arts-based approaches. The process involved in-depth discussions, not only with partner organisations, but also with young people, leading to a 'principle-based practice framework' grounded in lived experience, practitioner expertise, Mātauranga Māori (Māori knowledge), research, and evidence.

Gillian Howell's chapter examines participatory songwriting as an evaluative research method in humanitarian contexts, exploring its potential to centre adolescent voices and position young people as co-producers of knowledge. At the heart of the chapter is a step-by-step account of the development and implementation of the methodology for an international research and evaluation project, commissioned by Save the Children International's Middle East and Eastern Europe office. This account shows how the creative stages of participatory songwriting map onto the stages of a conventional research or evaluation process, but also how working with song can bring distinct benefits for the researchers/evaluators and participants. Ultimately, Howell argues that this approach provides a relational and non-extractive approach to learning about participants' perspectives.

Section 4: Arts as Evaluative Practices

Artistic and creative methods for evaluation are featured in chapters throughout this book. In this section, the chapters focus on the distinct features and affordances of arts-led or arts-based evaluation.

Linda Hassall and Natalie Lazaroo explore 'circus as method' to communicate migratory challenges faced by the endangered Far Eastern Curlew through the Climatescape project. Rather than conventional science communication approaches, the project investigated how embodied circus practices could creatively select, organise, and disseminate critical information about industrial and human mobility impacts on the Curlew's feeding and nesting behaviours. Key evaluation questions centred on whether circus could effectively communicate avian experiences, authentically enact more-than-human perspectives, and convey escalating global emergencies' impacts on local ecologies. The authors highlight circus's unique ability to transcend communication barriers through physical/visual expression while uniting written scholarship with embodied practice.

Kelly Freebody, Molly Mullen, Kim Snider, and Elise Sterback argue that a neoliberal ethos and related assumptions about individuals, bodies, and health are too often inadvertently taken up as the value system against which arts programmes are evaluated. To counter this, they draw on the ethico-political idea of the social flesh, developed by Chris Beasley and Carol Bacchi (2007), to explore how social embodiment might be taken more seriously in arts, health, and wellbeing evaluation. They share two examples of theatre and arts-based evaluative practices, which focused on concerns for collective wellbeing in particular contexts (a school and a local creative sector). Mobilising the concept of social flesh, the chapter considers how these examples open up possibilities for understanding and practising evaluation in ways that value embodied meaning-making and enact more equitable social relations.

Creating Conditions for Artful Evaluation

Our interest in artful, arts-based, and arts-led approaches to research and evaluation in the field of arts, health, and wellbeing reflects a shift in the scholarly discourse that draws together the different trends we discuss above. This shift is driven by a recognition of the limitations of traditional evaluation methods, which often struggle to capture the nuanced, subjective, and complex impacts of arts engagement on health and wellbeing. Scholars such as Veronica Baxter and Katharine Low (2017), Raw et al. (2012), and Tesch and Hansen (2013) argue that conventional quantitative and experimental research methods can be reductive and fail to fully represent the essence of the arts experience. In response, there is an increasing emphasis on embracing the aesthetic and affective dimensions of arts engagement, acknowledging the intrinsic value of the arts beyond their instrumental benefits for health (Baxter and Low 2017; Brodzinski 2010; Lafrenière et al. 2013; Simons and McCormick 2007). However, challenges remain in establishing the legitimacy and credibility of arts-based and other 'alternative' methods, particularly in the eyes of funders and commissioners who prioritise quantitative evidence (Baxter and Low 2017; Daykin et al. 2016). To address these challenges, scholars emphasise the need for transdisciplinary dialogue and the development of shared frameworks that bridge the perspectives, languages, and priorities of the arts and health sectors (Brodzinski 2010). Additionally, there is a strong emphasis on maintaining artistic quality and integrity in arts-based practices, cautioning against an overly instrumental view of the arts in health and wellbeing contexts (Brodzinski 2010; Baxter and Low 2017). As the field continues to evolve, artful approaches offer promising avenues for capturing the multifaceted impacts of arts engagement on health and wellbeing, while also presenting opportunities for more inclusive and meaningful evaluation practices.

References

Anderson, Michael., and O'Connor, Peter. 2014. Applied theatre as research: Provoking the possibilities. *Applied theatre research* 1(2): 189–202. https://doi.org/10.1386/atr.1.2.189_1

Ardern, Jacinda. 2018. Recognising the importance of our arts, culture and heritage. May 17. https://www.beehive.govt.nz/release/recognising-importance-our-arts-culture-and-heritage. Accessed 25 May 2025.

Arts Access Aotearoa. 2024. Te Kaha o ā Tatou maho – the power of our work: The impact of multi-year investment for creative spaces. https://cdn.fld.nz/uploads/sites/creativespaces/files/2025/Te_Kaha_report_files/Impact_of_multi-year_investment_for_creative_spaces_FINAL.pdf. Accessed 25 May 2025.

Australian Government. 2023. National Cultural Policy: Revive. https://www.arts.gov.au/publications/national-cultural-policy-revive-place-every-story-story-every-place. Accessed 25 May 2025.

Barclay, Leah. 2019. Acoustic ecology and ecological sound art: Listening to changing ecosystems. In *Sound, Media, Ecology,* eds. Milena Droumeva and Randolph Jordan, 153–177. London: Palgrave MacMillan

Bartleet, Brydie-Leigh, Naomi Sunderland, and Ali Lakhani. 2018. How can arts participation promote Indigenous social determinants of health?. In *Music, health and wellbeing: Exploring music for health equity and social justice*, ed. Naomi Sunderland, Natalie Lewandowski and Brydie-Leigh Bartleet, 201–226. London: Palgrave MacMillan.

Baxter, Veronica, and Katharine E. Low, eds. 2017. *Applied theatre: Performing health and wellbeing*. Bloomsbury Publishing.

Beasley, Chris, and Carol Bacchi. 2007. Beyond trust, care and generosity—towards an ethic of 'social flesh'. *Feminist Theory*, 8(3), 279–298.

Beck, Jaime. L., George Belliveau, Graham W. Lea, and Amanda Wager. 2011. Delineating a spectrum of research-based theatre. *Qualitative inquiry*, 17(8), 687–700. https://doi.org/10.1177/1077800411415498

Belfiore, Eleonora. 2015. 'Impact', 'value' and 'bad economics': Making sense of the problem of value in the arts and humanities. *Arts & Humanities in Higher Education* 14(1): 19–110. https://doi.org/10.1177/1474022214531503

Belfiore, Eleonora. 2020. Whose cultural value? Representation, power and creative industries. *International Journal of Cultural Policy* 26(3): 383–397. https://doi.org/10.1080/10286632.2018.1495713

Belfiore, Eleonora. 2022. Is it really about the evidence? argument, persuasion, and the power of ideas in cultural policy. *Cultural Trends* 31:4: 293–310. https://doi.org/10.1080/09548963.2021.1991230

Bhavnani, Kum-Kum. 1993. Tracing the contours: Feminist research and feminist objectivity. *Women's Studies International Forum* 16(2): 95–104. https://doi.org/10.1016/0277-5395(93)90001-P

Boydell, Katherine M., Michael Hodgins, Brenda M. Gladstone, Elaine Stasiulis, Geroge Belliveau, Hoi Cheu, Pia Kontos, and Janet Parsons. 2016. Arts-based health research and academic legitimacy: Transcending hegemonic conventions. *Qualitative Research* 16(6): 681–700. https://doi.org/10.1177/1468794116630040

Bright, Nicola, and Sally Boyd. 2024. Hei whakaarotanga: Engaging with models of health and wellbeing that draw on mātauranga Māori. NZCER Rangahau Mātauranga o Aotearoa. https://www.nzcer.org.nz/sites/default/files/downloads/Hei%20whakaarotanga%20-%20Engaging%20with%20models%20of%20health%20and%20wellbeing%20that%20draw%20on%20m%C4%81tauranga%20M%C4%81ori%20%28Full%20Report%29.pdf. Accessed 25 May 2025.

Brodzinski, Emma. 2010 *Theatre in health and care*. Springer.

Carr, Stuart. C., Jarrod Haar, James Liu, Sarah Kapeli, Darrin J. Hodgetts, Amanda Young-Hauser, Shiloh Groot, Mohi Rua, Rand Hazou, and Ahnya Martin. 2025. Linking wage to well-being: Subjectively experienced work precariousness. *International Perspectives in Psychology: Research, Practice, Consultation*. Advance online publication. https://doi.org/10.1027/2157-3891/a000112

Catalani, Caricia, and Meredith Minkler. 2010. Photovoice: A review of the literature in health and public health. *Health Education & Behavior* 37(3): 424–451. https://doi.org/10.1177/1090198109342084

Carter, Dave, Catherine Hoad, Paul Muller, Alice Tappenden, Jani Wilson, and Oli Wilson. 2024. Measuring and Articulating the Value of Live Performance in Aotearoa. Massey University. https://www.massey.ac.nz/documents/2119/Measuring-and-Articulating-the-Value-of-Live-Performance-in-Aotearoa.pdf. Accessed 25 May 2025.

Clift, Stephen, Kate Phillips, and Stephen Pritchard. 2021. The need for robust critique of research on social and health impacts of the arts. *Cultural Trends*, 30(5). 442–459. https://doi.org/10.1080/09548963.2021.1910492

Cole, Ardra L., and J. Gary Knowles. 2008. Arts-informed research. In *Handbook of the arts in qualitative research: Perspectives, methodologies, examples, and issues*, ed. J. Gary Knowles, 55–70. London: Sage.

Cooms, Samantha, and Vicki Saunders. 2024. Poetic inquiry: A tool for decolonising qualitative research. *Qualitative Research Journal* 24(1): 3–22. https://doi.org/10.1108/QRJ-05-2023-0071

Creative Australia. 2023. Creating Wellbeing: Attitudes and Engagement with Arts, Culture and Health. file:///C:/Users/mmul051/Downloads/Creating-Wellbeing-Report-2.pdf. Accessed 25 May 2025.

Creative Australia. 2025. Creative Australia backs new arts and health initiative to strengthen community connection. https://creative.gov.au/news-events/news/creative-Australia-backs-new-arts-and-health-initiative-strengthen-community. Accessed 6 November 2025.

Creative New Zealand. 2023. New Zealanders and the Arts—Ko Aotearoa me ōna Toi. https://creativenz.govt.nz/development-and-resources/new-zealanders-and-the-arts----ko-aotearoa-me-ona-toi. Accessed 25 May 2025.

Crossick, Geoffrey, and Patrycja Kaszynska. 2016. Understanding the value of arts and culture: The AHRC Cultural Value Project. Arts and Humanities Research Council. https://www.ukri.org/what-we-do/browse-our-areas-of-investment-and-support/ahrc-cultural-value-project/. Accessed 25 May 2025.

Daykin, Norma, Karen Gray, Mel McCree, and Jane Willis. 2017. Creative and credible evaluation for arts, health and well-being: Opportunities and challenges of co-production. *Arts and Health* 9, no. 2: 123–138. https://doi.org/10.1080/17533015.2016.1206948

Dudgeon, Pat, Abigail Bray, Dawn Darlaston-Jones, and Roz Walker 2020. Aboriginal Participatory Action Research: An Indigenous research methodology strengthening decolonisation and social and emotional wellbeing. Discussion Paper. Melbourne: The Lowitja Institute. https://www.lowitja.org.au/page/services/resources/Cultural-and-social-determinants/mental-health/aboriginal-participatory-action-research-an-indigenous-research-methodology-strengthening-decolonisation-and-social-and-emotional-wellbeing. Accessed 5 May 2025.

Durie, Mason. 2004. An indigenous model of health promotion. *Health Promotion Journal of Australia* 15(3): 181–185. https://doi.org/10.1071/HE04181

Ellis, Carolyn, Tony E. Adams, and Arthur P. Bochner. 2011. Autoethnography: An overview. *Historical Social Research/Historische Sozialforschung* 36(4): 273–290. http://www.jstor.org/stable/23032294

Forbes, Melissa, Genevieve A. Dingle, Nick Aitcheson, and Christa Powell. 2025. From Music Performance to Prescription: A Guide for Musicians and Health Professionals. *Music & Science*, *8*. https://doi.org/10.1177/20592043251338013

Freedland, Jonathan. 2007. Ministers seeking inspiration should talk to Pam about prewar Peckham. The Guardian, 31 October. https://www.theguardian.com/commentisfree/2007/oct/31/comment.politics1. Accessed 5 May 2025.

Gamble, Jamie. A. A. 2008. A developmental evaluation primer. The J.W. McConnell Family Foundation. https://mcconnellfoundation.ca/wp-content/uploads/2017/07/A-Developmental-Evaluation-Primer-EN.pdf. Accessed 25 May 2025.

Gattenhof, Sandra, Donna Hancox, Helen Klaebe, and Sasha Mackay. 2021. *The Social Impact of Creative Arts in Australian Communities*. 1st Edition 2021. Singapore: Springer. https://doi.org/10.1007/978-981-16-7357-3.

Gedutis, Aldis, Zoe Hope Bulaitis, and Michael Ochsner. 2023. The need for historical inquiry into societal impact evaluation: Towards a genealogy of the notion of useful research. In *Accountability in Academic Life: European Perspectives on Social Impact Evaluation*, eds. Michael Ochsner and Zoe Hope Bulaitis, 30–50. Edward Elgar Publishing.

Gee, Graham, Pat Dudgeon, Clinton Schultz, Amanda Hart, and Kerrie Kelly. 2014. Aboriginal and Torres Strait Islander social and emotional wellbeing. In *Working Together: Aboriginal and Torres Strait Islander Mental Health and Wellbeing Principles and Practice*, eds. Pat Dudgeon, Helen Milroy, and Roz Walker, 55–68. Canberra: Commonwealth of Australia.

Hardy, Pip, and Tony Sumner. 2017. Digital storytelling with users and survivors of the UK mental health system. In *Digital storytelling: Form and content*, edited by Mark Dunford and Tricia Jenkins, 57–69. Palgrave Macmillan.

Harriden, Kate. 2023. Working with Indigenous science(s) frameworks and methods: Challenging the ontological hegemony of 'western' science and the axiological biases of its practitioners. *Methodological Innovations* 16(2): 201–214. https://doi.org/10.1177/20597991231179394

Hickey, Sophie, Yvette Roe, Caroline Harvey, Sue Kruske, Anton Clifford-Motopi, Ike Fisher, Brenna Bernardino, and Sue Kildea. 2021. Community-Based Sexual and Reproductive Health Promotion and Services for First Nations People in Urban Australia. *International Journal of Women's Health* 13: 467–478. https://doi.org/10.2147/IJWH.S297479

House, Ernest R, and Kenneth R Howe. 1999. *Values in Evaluation and Social Research*. Thousand Oaks: Sage.

Kemmis, Stephen, and Robin McTaggart. 2005. *Participatory Action Research: Communicative Action and the Public Sphere*. In *The Sage handbook of qualitative research*, eds. Norman. K. Denzin and Yvonna. S. Lincoln, 559–603. London, Sage.

Lafrenière, Darquise, Susan M. Cox, George Belliveau, and Graham W. Lea. 2013. Performing the human subject: Arts-based knowledge dissemination in health research." *Journal of Applied Arts and Health* 3(3): 243–257. https://doi.org/10.1386/jaah.3.3.243_1

Leavy, Patricia. 2020. *Method meets art: Arts-based research practice*. London: The Guilford Press.

Matarasso, François. 2019. A Restless Art: How Participation Won, and Why it Matters. London, Calouste Gulbenkian Foundation.

McEwan, Alexandra, Alan Crouch, Heather Robertson, and Patricia Fagan. 2013. The Torres Indigenous Hip Hop Project: Evaluating the Use of

Performing Arts as a Medium for Sexual Health Promotion. *Health Promotion Journal of Australia* 24(2): 132–136. https://doi.org/10.1071/HE12924

McKegg, Kate, Nan Wehipeihana, M. Becroft, and J, Gill. 2016. Developmental Evaluation's Role in Supporting Community-Led Solutions for Māori and Pacific Young People's Educational Success: The Foundation North Māori and Pacific Education Initiative. In *Developmental evaluation exemplars: Principles in practice*, eds. Michael Quinn Patton, Kate McKegg and Nan Wehipeihana, 125–142. London: The Guildford Press.

Menezes, Stefanie. 2024. Virtual reality project healing Indigenous trauma receives $2.8m MRFF grant'. University of New South Wales: Newsroom. https://www.unsw.edu.au/newsroom/news/2024/10/VR-project-healing-indigenous-trauma-receives-2-8m-MRFF-grant. Accessed 5 May 2025.

Meyrick, Julian, Robert Phiddian, and Tully Barnett. 2018. *What matters?: talking value in Australian culture*. Melbourne: Monash University Publishing.

Morrow, Guy. 2022. Why Arts and Culture Appear to be the big Losers in this Budget. https://findanexpert.unimelb.edu.au/news/42187-why-arts-and-culture-appear-to-be-the-big-losers-in-this-budget. Accessed 25 May 2025.

Mullen, Molly, Amber Walls, Maria Ahmad, and Peter O'Connor. 2023. Resourcing the Arts for Youth Well-Being: Challenges in Aotearoa NZ. *Arts & Health* 15(1): 71–85. https://doi.org/10.1080/17533015.2021.2017306

Mullen, Molly, and Billie Lythberg. 2021. Kindness in Giving? Giving to and through the Arts in the Time of COVID-19. *Knowledge Cultures* 9(3): 111–38. https://www.ceeol.com/search/article-detail?id=999763

Nelson, Robin. 2013. *Practice as research in the arts: Principles, protocols, pedagogies, resistances*. London: Palgrave MacMillan.

Parr, Helen. 2017. Health and Arts: Critical Perspectives. In *Arts, Health and wellbeing: A theoretical inquiry for practice, eds.* Theo Stickley and Stephen Clift: 14–23. Newcastle upon Tyne: Cambridge Scholars Publishing.

Patton, Michael Quinn. 2011. *Developmental evaluation: Applying complexity concepts to enhance innovation and use*. London: The Guilford Press.

Patton, Michael Quinn. 2023. Public policy evaluation: origins and evolution. In *Handbook of Public Policy Evaluation*, eds. Frédéric Varone, Steve Jacob, and Pirmin Bundi, 16–30. Edward Elgar Publishing.

Prendergast, Monica, Carl Leggo, and Pauline Sameshima. 2009. *Poetic inquiry: Vibrant voices in the social sciences*. Rotterdam: Sense Publishers.

Prendergast, Monica, Juliana Saxton, and Yasmine Kandil. 2024. *Applied theatre: International case studies and challenges for practice*. Intellect Books.

Raw, Annie, Sue Lewis, Andrew Russell, and Jane Macnaughton. 2012. A hole in the heart: Confronting the drive for evidence-based impact research in arts and health. *Arts & Health*, 4(2): 97–108. https://doi.org/10.1080/17533015.2011.619991

Roy, Eleanor. 2019. New Zealand's world-first 'wellbeing' budget to focus on poverty and mental health. The Guardian, 14 May. https://www.theguardian.com/world/2019/may/14/new-zealands-world-first-wellbeing-budget-to-focus-on-poverty-and-mental-health. Accessed 5 May 2025.

Saldaña, Johnny. 2011. *Ethnotheatre: Research from page to stage*. Left Coast Press.

Simons, Helen, and Brendan McCormack. 2007. Integrating arts-based inquiry in evaluation methodology: Opportunities and challenges. *Qualitative inquiry* 13(2): 292–311. https://doi.org/10.1177/1077800406295622

Sunderland, Naomi, Phil Graham, Brydie-Leigh Bartleet, Darren Garvey, Clint Bracknell, Kristy Apps, Glenn Barry, Rae Cooper, Brigitta Scarfe, and Stacey Vervoort. 2023. First Nations music as a determinant of health in Australia and Vanuatu: political and economic determinants. *Health Promotion International* 38(2): 190. https://doi.org/10.1093/heapro/daac190

Sunderland, Naomi, Natalie Lewandowski, Dan Bendrups, and Brydie-Leigh Bartleet, eds. 2018. *Music, Health and Wellbeing: Exploring Music for Health Equity and Social Justice*. Palgrave Macmillan. https://research.ebsco.com/linkprocessor/plink?id=1696518d-5caa-3cd9-a082-2d0b79bce1ea.

Smith, Linda Tuhiwai. 2012. *Decolonizing Methodologies: Research and Indigenous Peoples*. London, UK: Zed Books.

Snyder-Young, Dani, Michael Arnold Mages, Rahul Bhargava, Jonathan Carr, Laura Perovich, Victor Talmadge, Oliver Wason, Moira Zellner, Angelique C-Dina, Ren Birnholz, and et al. 2024. Viewpoints/Points of View: Building a Transdisciplinary Data Theatre Collaboration in Six Scenes. *Arts* 13(1): 37. https://doi.org/10.3390/arts13010037

Tesch, Leigh, and Emily C. Hansen. 2013. Evaluating effectiveness of arts and health programmes in primary health care: A descriptive review. *Arts & Health* 5(1): 19–38. https://doi.org/10.1080/17533015.2012.693512

Van Styvendale, Nancy, J. D. McDougall, Robert Henry, and Robert Alexander Innes. 2021. *The arts of Indigenous health and well-being*. University of Manitoba Press

Verbunt, Ebony, Joanne Luke, Yin Paradies, Muriel Bamblett, Connie Salamone, Amanda Jones, and Margaret Kelaher. 2021. Cultural Determinants of Health for Aboriginal and Torres Strait Islander People–a Narrative Overview of Reviews. *International Journal for Equity in Health* 20: 1–9. https://link.springer.com/article/10.1186/s12939-021-01514-2

Vincent, James. 2023. *Beyond Measure: The hidden history of measurement*. London: Faber and Faber.

Walls, Amber. 2023. Activating the Arts for Youth Wellbeing in Aotearoa: Practices, Principles and Possibilities [Doctoral Thesis]. New Zealand: University of Auckland.

Woodland, Sarah, Kamarra Bell-Wykes, and THE SCORE Ensemble. 2024. THE SCORE: Participatory theatre for sexual health education in First Nations Communities. AIATSIS Report. University of Melbourne and Ilibjerri Theatre Company. https://www.ilbijerri.com.au/event/thescore/. Accessed 25 May 2025.

World Health Organisation. 2025. World report on social determinants of health equity 2025. https://www.who.int/news/item/06-05-2025-health-inequities-are-shortening-lives-by-decades. Accessed 25 May 2025.

Zamenopoulos, Theodore, and Katerina Alexiou. 2018. *Co-design as Collaborative* Research. Bristol University/AHRC Connected Communities Programme. https://oro.open.ac.uk/58301/

PART I

What is of Value

CHAPTER 2

What Is of Value in the Learning Disabled Theatre of Different Light?

Tony McCaffrey

Introduction: Mary Miller and the Value of Disabled Performance

I recently attended a screening of *Two Minutes of Ordinary Everyday Life* (2024). The film by Many Hats, a Christchurch-based disability performance group, caused me to re-assess what I mean by the value of disability performance. It also forced me to consider how participants in such projects might value their experience of the making of and dissemination of performance that draws so deeply on their lived experience. It also encouraged me to question the evaluation of the aesthetic and political efficacy or impact of disability performance that far too often is based on a mechanistic model of input and output, of profit and loss (Fig. 2.1).

In one scene, viewers are introduced to Mary Miller, a woman with cerebral palsy who uses a motorised wheelchair and lives in a retirement home in Ōtautahi Christchurch, Aotearoa New Zealand. She is also a

T. McCaffrey (✉)
National Academy of Singing and Dramatic Art, Ara Institute, Christchurch, New Zealand
e-mail: tony.mccaffrey@ara.ac.nz

M. Mullen et al. (eds.), *Artful Evaluation for Creative Health and Wellbeing*, New Directions in Cultural Policy Research,
https://doi.org/10.1007/978-3-032-17063-7_2

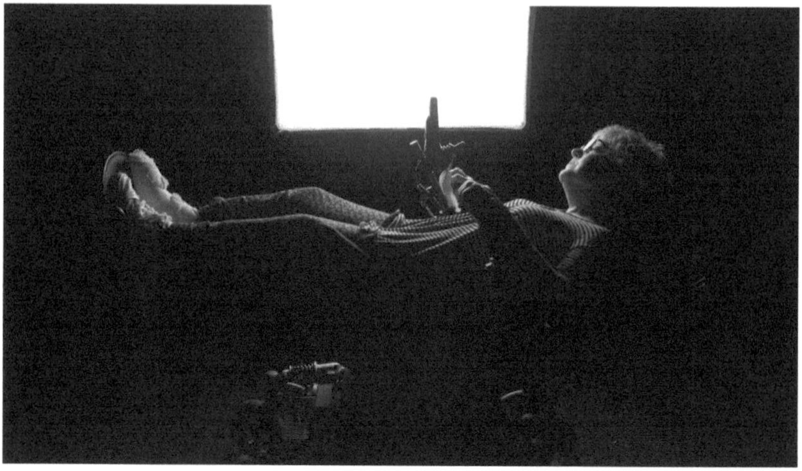

Fig. 2.1 An image of Mary Miller from the film *Two Minutes of Ordinary Everyday Life*. Image by Paul McCaffrey (2024)

member of disability performance group Many Hats. When she was asked what aspect of her ordinary life she wanted to be filmed, she chose the event of getting out of bed. Miller uses a remote to lower the bed. To get up off the bed, she has to negotiate the movement of her body with the help of an assistive device. In the film, we see her repeated and faltering efforts to get up off the bed and into the gutter walking frame. This takes several minutes, all while Miller talks to the camera. She talks us through the elaborate process of her movements to achieve what would be a simple action for a non-disabled person. Miller's physical inhabiting of the world shrinks to her body's hard won but small victories in eventually raising herself onto the walking frame, her persistence in accomplishing her movements despite not being able to feel the floor, her negotiation of the three point turn, and her finally sitting in the chair. Her morning routine, and her life as a whole, is subject to what Arseli Dokumaci (2023) terms the 'shrinkage' of chronic pain and debility 'the constraints, failures and losses' of impairment, the intransigence of her disability to allow her to cope with any sense of ease in the spatiotemporal environment. And yet something else emerges in Miller's daily struggle. To quote Dokumaci:

> As actors relate to the stage and its props within the imaginative layer of performance, they transform this materiality into an elsewhere and an elsewhen through their actions. I argue that the same transformation takes place in the everyday lives of disabled people, which are lived within a shrinking world of possibilities [...] when the world's offerings become unreachable in states of extreme deprivation and debilitation, it is exactly the imaginary space of performance that opens up. (2023, 8)

What might be the value of this performance? What conceptions of value are opened up by this performance? What might be the value of this performance for Mary Miller? If she wishes to get up in the morning, this performance is an integral part of her life. What is the value of the making of the film to her? She wants people to understand what her everyday, ordinary life entails and the performance she undergoes to have her everyday ordinary life. Her life and the affordances she creates to render the world more habitable can only happen if she pays attention to the diverse needs of her body in relation to the environment, human and non-human, of which she is a part.

There are various models of evaluation that could apply to Mary Miller's performance of her 'five minutes of ordinary everyday life'. She is a remarkable example of resilience in the face of debilitating disability; she is succeeding in improvising creative affordances in the face of an ableist world. These are undoubtedly fair evaluations to a certain extent. What cannot be gainsaid, however, is the intractability of her disability, the limitations of impairment which need to be faced, accepted, and challenged daily. In the daily struggles, the scant victories of Mary Miller we need to acknowledge both the intransigence and the hard-won beauty and dignity of disability in performance.

I would now like to discuss some recent examples of performance and the various forms of evaluation that are at play in disability performance from my own experience with my learning disabled co-researchers of Different Light Theatre. We have been co-researching the possibilities of learning-disabled theatre for twenty years. The power dynamic in this relationship needs to be acknowledged: my position as non-disabled director and facilitator is vastly different in terms of privilege and acknowledgement to my learning disabled colleagues. This discussion will be, in effect, a consideration of who values what. This includes the evaluation of the performers, me as a non-disabled director/researcher, participants in the field of academic conferences and publications and the funders and other organisations that enable the continuing participation of Different Light Theatre in public performances and presentations at academic conferences. This consideration of the different conceptions and practices of evaluation includes an analysis of the contribution made by the learning disabled performers/researchers of Different Light to the Performance Philosophy Problems conference held in 2022 in Helsinki and online. It also includes the response by the group to questions raised about their presence at this conference. This response was to create another performance at the University of Auckland in 2023.

What follows is a consideration of the different kinds of value that might be ascribed to the group's activities and how such values might be assessed. I consider these questions within this piece of writing, but my contention is that my learning disabled collaborators also consider these same questions from their perspective: from their lived experience of devising, collaboration, performance and engagement with audiences and of travelling while disabled in an ableist world. My writing voice is dominant here, but I hope it resonates with the shared experiences of twenty years of collaboration in the Different Light project. Perhaps the main value of this project is in its attempt to listen the voices of the learning disabled performers into speech.

Should Learning Disabled Theatre be Valued in Terms of an Economy or an Ecosystem?

DJ Savarese is a nonverbal public speaker, writer and activist who communicates through a voice synthesiser. He states the following about autistics' prioritising of the sensory over the verbal: 'We feel ourselves less as citizens of a domain, and more as interdependent beings within a vast ecosystem' (2024, 1). Savarese goes on to connect this highly political shift in perception in terms that are framed in the language of evaluation:

> I remind typical people...that their prized sense of normalcy comes at a cost. A cost exacted not just from them, but from every other being within our ecosystem. Such a rational distant-I cannot grasp that we are all made up of matter and so must care for each other. (ibid)

As a poet, Savarese's choice of words is significant. The normalcy of neurotypical people is 'prized'—of superior value—yet this privilege comes at a cost. This is a cost that the bearer of the privilege cannot on their own hope to pay as it is a cost exacted from the whole ecosystem in which 'they' and 'we' operate.

What Savarese's sentences also illustrate is how much our language of evaluation is caught up in economic meanings of value. If I ask what value disability performance has or even if I try to reconfigure what is meant by the value of such activity, I am caught up in the very lexis and syntax of input and output, of profit and loss that renders it very difficult to express or articulate alternative relationships or processes. What value, efficacy, or use does disability performance have? What would happen if we were to temper economically based evaluation with an acknowledgement of the mutual inter-relationships of ecosystems? Where does such speculation go? What is the use of such speculation to the people involved? Do we need to re-evaluate the concept of 'use' as is indicated by a trend in recent critical theory in feminist and disability studies to validate what is conventionally termed 'useless'?

Sara Ahmed's *What's the Use? On the Uses of Use* (2019) and Erin Manning's *For a Pragmatics of the Useless?* (2020) are useful examples of scholarship probing questions of use. In terms of learning-disabled theatre specifically, there is a great desire amongst funders and support organisations to 'instrumentalise' theatre to *make use of* theatre to heal perceived rifts in the social bond, to *apply* theatre as if it were a panacea for diversity, equity, and inclusion. At the end of his introduction to Matt Hargrave's *Theatres of Learning Disability: Good, Bad, or Plain Ugly?* Tim Wheeler, former Artistic Director of renowned UK learning-disabled theatre company Mind the Gap, refers to his hope in moving beyond the 'applied theatre' model:

> My hope for the future is that we are able to make the case for a dis-applied theatre. Not as a replacement for the excellent work done within the applied theatre framework but as an option that can, if appropriate, remove the obligation to make theatre with learning disabled people to cure or console. (Cited in Hargrave 2015, 8)

Different Light and the Performance Philosophy Problems Project

In 2021, Different Light Theatre took part in a Key Group Presentation for the conference 'Performance Philosophy Problems: How Does Performance Philosophy Collaborate?' at the University of the Arts in Helsinki. The conference was originally scheduled for June 2021 but postponed due to the COVID-19 pandemic and was hosted as a hybrid iteration in June 2022. The other members of the Key Group 'Collaboration, Conviviality and Care' were Dave Calvert from University of Huddersfield, Kate Maguire-Rosier from University of New South Wales, and Janet Gibson from University of Sydney. The Different Light performers and I presented on how we collaborate in performance, presentations, and publication. The intention of this participation was from my perspective, an attempt to include the voice and presence of learning-disabled performers in academic discourse and research. It was an attempt both to facilitate and problematise that voice and presence.

In preparation for the presentation, eight to ten members of Different Light Theatre and I regularly met on Zoom during the lockdowns of the COVID-19 pandemic. After years of in-person rehearsals and meetings this enforced method of collaboration impressed upon us the importance of being together even in a reconfigured and somewhat restricted form. The regularity and reliability of meeting at the same time with the same people were something that all of us could hold onto in the face of the vagaries, fears, and isolations of the lockdowns. This virtual co-presence alerted us to the value of what we were trying to hold onto: the sense of conviviality that had developed after years of being together. The value of this project for those of us as academics/practitioners was in the attempt to include learning-disabled participants who were usually the subjects of research rather than the makers or doers of research.

The Interview Effect

The value for the performers of participation in the conference and related activities is harder to gauge. One obvious method of evaluation might be simply to ask the learning-disabled performers what was valuable to them in this project. My experience, however, is that the overt asking of questions of value to learning disabled performers in a kind of social science model of research is not likely to achieve anything more than an agreement that such activities are of value. In *Giving and Taking Voice in Learning Disabled Theatre* (2023), I have written about the 'interview effect' in researching learning-disabled theatre, in which:

> The imperative to conduct 'social science' type interviews or to demand an account of experience and subjectivity is itself fraught with the oppressive dynamics of power manifest in interpellation, the kairotic time of the interview itself and the tendency of the interviewee to assimilate to, appease, or please the interviewer. (McCaffrey, 12)

In the face of this effect, at Different Light we have tried to devise different strategies to afford the emergence of the voices of the performers. These include:

- the use of performer-led interviews, often using video, to turn the 'expected' interview relationship on its head.
- discursive strategies of conversation, or the intertwining of different conversations to render any 'interview' less explicitly goal oriented.
- maintaining a constant awareness of what is going on in the room
- drawing on the ethics of attunement of Lisbeth Lipari: 'a listening others to speech that can reverse authoritative normative social arrangements that [...] silence others and refuse to listen' (2014, 95).

These emergent strategies and tangential processes were reflected in the text that was generated by the Different Light performers for the video presentation sent to the Helsinki conference in 2022. I presented the performers with some basic information about the conference, the location, the people involved, and the theme of the conference. They then responded to this basic information as they chose. In addition, we as a group tried to stay close to what was going on in our times together (online and in person) at that period. I reproduce the entire transcript of the curated video message below:

JOSIE AND BIDDY:	Hello, Helsinki!
ANGIE (coming onstage in her wheelchair):	Hello, Helsinki!
JOSIE and BIDDY: (running on behind her):	Hello, Helsinki!

MATTHEW P:	Tahi, Rua, Toru, Whā[1]
ALL:	Hello Helsinki! Hei Helsinki!
DAMIAN:	How can we get to Helsinki? How can we do that?
BIDDY:	We can communicate with you via Zoom
PETER:	(On Zoom) Welcome to Performance Philosophy Problems
ALL:	Welcome
MATTHEW S:	Haere mai, haere mai, haere mai[2]
MATTHEW P:	What are Performance Philosophy Problems?
JOSIE:	We are Performance Philosophy Problems
PETER:	No you are
ALL:	You are. No you are. You are
BIDDY:	Guys focus, please stay focussed
MATTHEW P:	We are Different Light Theatre, a theatre group from Christchurch New Zealand
PETER:	We've been through earthquakes
ANGIE:	Floods, massacres
MATTHEW S:	Fires,
JOSIE:	Viruses, a global pandemic
ANGIE:	Lockdowns, isolations
BIDDY:	Anti-mandate protests
ISAAC:	And a war in Ukraine
DAMIAN:	And now Isaac's poem…
ISAAC:	So much depends on my support workers, So much depends on vaccination, So much depends on police, So much depends on our lives matter, so much depends on thinking
MATTHEW P:	NOW WE ARE GOING TO ASK YOU SOME QUESTIONS
BIDDY:	FOR OUR RESEARCH
JOSIE:	Please answer them to the best of your ability
PETER:	Number 1.What is your disability?
ISAAC:	Number 2.Who are your caregivers?

[1] Māori for 'One, Two, Three, Four'.

[2] Māori greeting or welcome.

ANGIE:	Number 3. How do you get in and out of bed?
MATTHEW P:	Unfortunately, we don't have any time for your answers
JOSIE:	You will need to take your answers away with you
ANGIE:	I try to talk to people all the time and they just walk away. By the way, I use a hoist to get in and out of bed
PETER:	Question 4. Why did the person in a motorised wheelchair cross the road?
MATTHEW P:	How can the person in a motorised wheelchair cross the road?
BIDDY:	Hei, Esa Kirkkopelto!
ALL:	Hei, Esa!
PETER:	Esa told us we need to do something like a performance but we can rehearse it
BIDDY:	I think Esa looks like a professional and he looks like he has been doing this for a while
MATTHEW P:	I've been doing theatre for a while
JOSIE AND OTHERS:	I have too. ME TOO. AND ME
JOSIE:	The last public performance we did was The History of Different Light for the Christchurch Arts Festival in 2019
ISAAC:	Since then we have had to rethink what we mean by performance…
MATTHEW S:	We can make theatre together
ISAAC:	… and thinking
ANGIE:	Right now
JOSIE:	We are in an Omicron surge here in Christchurch
MATTHEW P:	To protect ourselves and others we need to meet on Zoom
PETER:	On Zoom you can talk to your mates
ANGIE:	You can laugh with them
BIDDY:	You can use filters or share screen (Heart filters appear around her)
JOSIE:	On Zoom you can't be with them in person
MATTHEW P AND GLEN:	You can't hug them
ANGIE AND JOSIE AND OTHERS:	You can't drink coffee with them and share a meal with them
MATTHEW P:	The question is: Can you do theatre on Zoom?

ISAAC: The question is: Can you do thinking on Zoom? (Gibson et al. 2024, 1–2)

This is a document of the processes of the group at that time. I believe it gives evidence of what both the learning disabled performers valued and I valued (values that both overlapped and were distinct) in what we were doing as we presented ourselves on the virtual stage of the Performance Philosophy conference. The contributions from the performers emphasised connection—both with those organising and attending the conference and with each other through the isolations and virtual connections of the lockdowns. Greetings and welcomes were valued, as was some basic recognition of tangata whenua (te reo Māori for the people of the land) of the ground on which they were speaking. I approached the participation of the Different Light performers in the academic conference as important in terms of having some representation of learning disabled performers/researchers in that academic space. The performers themselves, on the other hand, approached the event differently.

What is the Performance Philosophy of Different Light?

In order to articulate that difference I need to give a context for the basic concepts of 'performance' and 'philosophy' that might be said to constitute the epistemology of Different Light. 'Performance' or the changing meanings of what performance means to the group was a subject we had been investigating amongst ourselves for a number of years. This practice had ranged from our initial attempts at naïve community theatre to attempts to present dramatic theatre for public performance, to post-dramatic, site-specific experimentation, collaboration in performance art events and performance and attendance at a number of academic conferences. One thing performance did not consistently mean for the members of the company was paid or 'gainful' employment. We have in the past received Creative New Zealand funding for tours to Australia, the United States and the United Kingdom but these mainly covered costs of travel, accommodation, and providing the basic technology of theatrical performance. Any box office revenue from performances has gone towards the creation of future projects.

In speaking of the evaluation of the work of Different Light Theatre, it needs to be stated that there has never been a period in which the performers have regularly received sustainable financial recompense for their labour. In addition, despite participation in performances, presentations and continuing research, the performers have never, as yet, received any qualifications or institutional recognition of their work. After twenty years, it is possible to say that the group exists on the principle of whanaungatanga (relationships) and in effect in an economy of koha (gift). If conditions were right, however, the group certainly would want to be valued professionally and educationally. At the same time, I do not want to denigrate the bonds of love, obligation, commitment, and mutual care that inform the groups continuing to be together and research into what it means to be together.

What 'philosophy' means to the group is more difficult to ascertain and needs to be approached in quite discursive and diverse ways. The ethos of the group is always to be inclusive; to find ways of including whoever wants to be a member of the group. This has extended to hospital and home visits when people were unable to attend the regular weekly devising and rehearsal sessions, and, latterly, online participation, when possible. We have thus far always been able to find funding sources to allow all those who wanted to participate in performance and touring. A commitment to telling the stories of the disabled performers has emerged over time but this has never been at the expense of the chance to play or experiment with broadly theatrical *ways of telling*.

The philosophy of the members of Different Light, if such a thing exists, is composed of a commitment to self-expression. But the 'self' of individual members of the company is problematic and elusive given the marginalised access to systems of expression and communication concomitant with a diagnosis of intellectual disability. If there were a 'self' of the company as an organic entity, it would be likewise elusive and 'content not to be a single being' to reconfigure the quote by Édouard Glissant (2011, 5).

This very loose philosophy of the company was summed up in a simple phrase devised by performer Isaac Tait for the contribution to the Performance Philosophy Problems conference: 'We are performance philosophy problems'. Learning disabled people are performance philosophy problems as they are not considered as philosophical subjects or they constitute an ethical problem, in the sense that learning disabled people are subjected to ethics rather than ever being treated as ethical subjects.

In the supposedly more academic paper that I gave following the video message that the group presented at this conference, I attempted to riff on the material the performers had devised. This was a transitional strategy to try to acknowledge the contributions of the learning disabled performers by intertwining their devised text and responses within a more conventional academic discourse. This was an attempt to contextualise the participation of the performers and to acknowledge the 'thinking' that goes on in the devising and rehearsal room, what Margaret Ames and her learning disabled co-researchers call 'thinking no-one's thought' (Ames 2019, 299). This thinking is manifest in what I would term the emergent ecosystems of collaboration, care and conviviality that constitute the twenty years' experience of Different Light Theatre. The past few years of the company's operation and the turn to research have been in a way a quest for understanding and experiencing the value of what we can do together and of what value this might have for others. Learning disabled and neurodivergent artists should be valued. This valuation encompasses at a basic level the right to exist, the right to recompense for labour, the right to be considered as artists in their own right: possessed of the ability to speak to others in languages that may not be understood in the same ways as neurotypical lines of communication, and possessed of the ability to create beauty that deviates from norms of spatiality and temporality.

What is of value in the form and understanding of theatre that I have tried to give or to share with the learning disabled artists of Different Light over twenty years? This is a salutary question. For twenty years, I have been a fellow traveller, I have briefly shared with learning disabled artists journeys to theatrical performance, academic conferences, international Zoom presentations, to appearances and disappearances, to hospitals, to birthdays, and, in two instances, to the end of life. We started the company in 2004 based on my understanding of theatre. In this understanding, so much depended on resonant voices, so much depended on engaged and articulate bodies. This particular understanding of theatre then came into contact with the learning-disabled artists.

It has taken me twenty years to listen, if only a little, to try to attend and attune to learning disabled people. In 2004, I invited the learning-disabled artists to theatre. I gave 'theatre' to them. In the paradox of hospitality and hostility traced by Derrida, in giving them theatre I not only short changed them on what theatre might mean but I also gave them the bonds of obligation. In *Monolingualism of the Other*, Derrida starkly presents the hostility underlying the values of forgiving, giving and inviting:

> At bottom, nothing is more vulgar and impolite, even wounding, than to obligate someone by telling them 'I forgive you' which implies an 'I give you' and already opens a scene of acknowledgement (reconnaissance), a transaction of gratitude, a commerce of thinking that destroys the gift. Similarly, one must never say 'I grant you hospitality' or 'I invite you'. When one says 'I invite you' it means: I pay and we are inscribed in the circular commerce of the most inhospitable exchange possible, the least giving. (1998, 398)

This notion of 'giving' hospitality underpinned by hostility for me inflects the development of much learning-disabled theatre and the charity, therapeutic or socially engaged imperatives of the form from the 1980s onwards.

Learning disabled artists make for uneasy guests, uneasier hosts in the academy, at the conference, at the symposium, and in the spaces of making theatre. Every week ten of us, two in motorised wheelchairs, follow our customary lines to take a break from devising and rehearsal. To get to the café we cross a six-lane road with two sets of traffic lights. They are on timers. Green man. Red man flashing. Beepbeepbeepbeep. Traffic revving. Red man. Zoom. They're off. There is never enough time. Why would a person in a motorised wheelchair want to cross the road? Who are your caregivers? How do you get in and out of bed? On Zoom we talk over each other, miss turns, look at ourselves, cannot feel the nonverbal cues of the person responding, the slight delay, the freeze, the microphone disabled. What of the zoomtime of necro-capitalism and the Socio-Ecological Disaster, can we do theatre, can we do thinking in this zoomtime?

After the KeyGroup Presentation at the Helsinki conference in the question-and-answer session at which members of Different Light were present online, Laura Cull O Maoilearca asked a crucial question addressing many of the concerns about the place and value of both learning disabled artists and the academic conference:

> I'm thinking about how the presentation from Different Light and their presence their withusness makes an academic paper look and feel...I'm asking it as someone who also gives academic papers and is struggling to think and understand why we do that, why we still do this, and how we

> can be together in conferences in meaningful and inclusive ways. I'm not asking because I think I know something, but it's impossible to get away from the resonance of that phrase 'nothing about us without us' How do we do that? What is 'aboutness' What is 'withusness'? (Gibson et al. 1)

Different Light Theatre responded to Cull Ó Maoilearca's questions with a performance. The group's participation at the Helsinki conference was at a distance geographically, temporally and mediated through technology. For the next project, Different Light gave a performance in real life with an audience present, *The Journeyings of Different Light*, at 'Travelling Together' the conference of the Australasian Association for Theatre, Drama, and Performance Studies at the University of Auckland, Aotearoa New Zealand, 6–9 December 2022. My motivation was both to maintain a research profile for myself and the group and to afford the performers an opportunity to travel and to engage again in in-person performance for the first time in three years.

Angelia Douglas and the Auckland Performance

Collectively, we made a commitment to proceed with the Auckland performance. I raised funds from the Ara Foundation to cover the costs of flights and accommodation for eight performers. We negotiated the 'necessary' risk assessments for certain performers, we obtained permission for travel from performers' EPOAs (Enduring Power of Attorney), we organised two support people to accompany the performers and me. Angelia Douglas's support people organised a manual wheelchair—to traverse the steep gradients of busy Auckland roads rather than relying on her motorised wheelchair that was guided sometimes erratically by the little finger of her right hand and a hoist—for getting her in and out of bed. This was her first time out of the South Island of Aotearoa New Zealand, her first time travelling in an aeroplane. The airline managed to damage both wheelchair and hoist in ways that severely impacted her mobility and comfort. A performer tripped and fainted at Auckland airport. Another performer vomited backstage just before the performance. We experienced the 'performances around performance' of disability performance. There is a colloquial phrase in English 'What a performance!' that is used in the context that the Oxford English Dictionary defines as 'a difficult, time-consuming or annoying action or procedure'; this is often the kind of performance that accompanies the access of disabled artists to theatrical performance.

In one of the rehearsals in Auckland, Angelia Douglas really struggled to maintain her posture due to the right arm of her manual chair being unusable as a result of being damaged in transit. Noting this, Josie Noble, for large parts of the rehearsal, found a way of moving and supporting Douglas' right arm and leading her through the movements of the simple dance sequences. When we returned to Ōtautahi Christchurch, we discovered that she was covered in bruises from the ups and downs of Auckland pavements and her lack of familiarity with travelling any distance in a manual wheelchair. This was a salutary lesson. I had imagined that I was offering Douglas an experience that would be of value to her: her first time out of the South Island, first time in an aeroplane and first time in Auckland. She did remarkably well in her first public performance and also participated meaningfully in the conference, but I had not reckoned with the physical and emotional cost to her of this valuable experience.

We know more now in hindsight, of course, and despite this and numerous other difficulties, she has persisted in working with the company, including in October 2023 on the collaboration with eighteen drama school students on a production of *Faust.Us* loosely based on Marlowe's Renaissance English text. In one section of that performance, she was required in the persona of one of Faustus' good angels to speak some lines about a moment she valued in her life in order to convince Faustus to repent and pursue the path of goodness. The words she chose were: 'In Kaikoura I watch the whales surface in the van with my Mum', She was, however, very rarely able to complete the speaking of these lines without crying.

It was not until much later that she was able to offer a verbal explanation for this behaviour. This was when Different Light was working on a new and separate project, Ancient Greek Theatre and Intellectual Disability, an international collaboration with learning disabled theatre companies in Australia, Belgium, Greece, Poland, Switzerland and the UK, leading to a proposed festival of learning-disabled theatre in 2025/6. In a rehearsal for this project, she devised the following text:

> When I act I am a totally different person. Because it makes me feel like I don't have a wheelchair, when I act with Different Light. When I talk about my family history there is a story I need to tell. When I was with my birth mum Joy she was a person of many talents but one day a tragedy

> happened in the family. The whole family knew about this until this day came. I went to see my birth mum she wasn't very well on this day which my feelings became real when I heard my stepdad on the phone to the ambulance people which then they came in to the house and said What can we do for you? My dad said I think Joy became very unwell which led her to go to hospital and they discovered that she had terminal cancer. (Douglas, 2024)

She also subsequently sent a photograph of her younger self sitting with her Māori birth mother (Fig. 2.2).

She went on to describe the significance of the picture in her devised text:

> This is my mom when we were living in 11 karo place in Ilam. Well I was at Laura Fergusson early on I my life. Here is a photo you will find attached to the rest of the book that I want you to help with (p.s. You have got my brain working overtime, which means I will think of anything I do from now on). This is the end of what you and I wrote this morning. You can attach to it, if you can. If you can't, we will work on it on Sunday. I like telling people how I feel by words, not by voice, cause then I can I be my normal self. With you and Different Light.

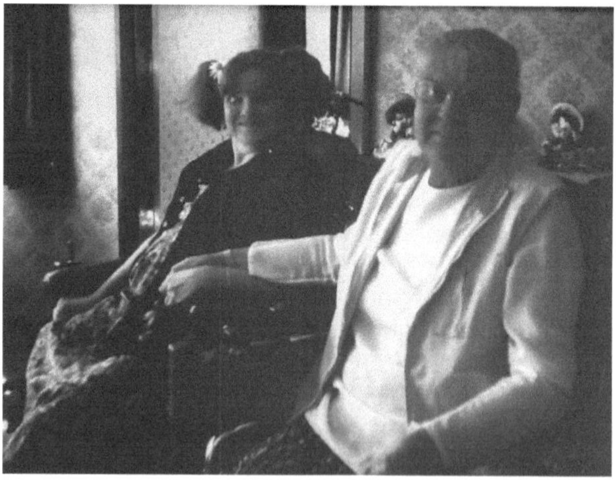

Fig. 2.2 An image of Angie sitting with her Māori birth mother. Image by Angelia Douglas (n.d.)

> This was a day before she got terminally ill.
> This gives you and the rest of the crew some idea of what my upbringing was like. That is why I get quite sad when I am acting because I am thinking about her at the same time of me trying to act. So you can attach it to this morning's work from me. It was nice of Issac to help me today. As I know Issac was not feeling the best but he was there for me. (Douglas 2024)

What is clear to me from Douglas' contribution to the present piece of writing is that she does value her participation in the theatre making of Different Light but it is a value that comes at a cost to her. In terms of the trip to Auckland and regular attendance at rehearsals, this cost is a drain on her stamina. In terms of her investment in the representative mechanisms of theatre and the testimonial aspects of narrative, this cost is emotional: an encounter with longing, desire and regret that can at times be painful. The second book that has arisen out of the work of the company contains 90,000 words, 20,000 of which are directly attributable to the learning disabled members of the company, collated and curated through a range of different strategies. The title is *Giving and Taking Voice in Learning Disabled Theatre* (2023). Angelia Douglas' experience aligns with the duality of this title. Making theatre, giving voice, putting your 'self' out there as a performance persona gives you the possibility of expression and imagining other selves. It also takes something from you. Perhaps the real value of learning-disabled theatre is in the acceptance of this shimmering back and forth between presence and loss.

References

Ahmed, Sara. 2019. *What's the Use? On the Uses of Use*. Durham: Duke University Press.

Ames, Margaret. 2019. Learning Disability, Thought, and Theatre. *Contemporary Theatre Review* 29. 3: 290–304.

Calvert, Dave, Kate Maguire-Rosier, Janet Gibson, Tony McCaffrey, and Different Light Theatre. 2022. Collaboration, Conviviality and Care: The Problem of Including Learning-Disabled and Neurodivergent Artists in Performance Philosophy. Paper presented at *Performance Philosophy Problems* Conference, University of the Arts, Helsinki and online. 15–18 June.

Derrida, Jacques. 1998. *Monolingualism of the Other or the Prosthesis of Origin*. Transl. Patrick Mensah. Stanford: Stanford University Press.

Dokumaci, Arseli. 2023. *Activist Affordances: How Disabled People Improvise More Habitable Worlds*. Durham: Duke University Press.

Douglas, Angelia. 2024. Unpublished rehearsal transcripts. March 21–28.

Faust.Us. 2023. Different Light Theatre and NASDA. Directed by Tony McCaffrey. NASDA Theatre, Christchurch, 10–16 Nov.

Two Minutes of Ordinary Everyday Life, directed by Paul McCaffrey. (Many Hats Theatre and Film, 2024).

Gibson, Janet, Kate Maguire-Rosier, and Tony McCaffrey. 2024. 'We are Performance Philosophy Problems': Towards an accessible performance philosophy? *Performance Philosophy Journal* 9.1. https://performancephilosophy.org/journal/article/view/443

Glissant, Édouard. 2011. One World in Relation: Édouard Glissant in conversation with Manthia Diawara. Translated by C. Winks. *Nka Journal of Contemporary African Art* 28 (Spring): 4–19. https://doi.org/10.1215/10757163-1266639

Hargrave, Matt. 2015. *Theatres of learning disability: Good, bad, or plain ugly?* Basingstoke: Palgrave Macmillan.

Lipari, Lisbeth. 2014. Ethics, kairos and akroasis: An essay on time and relation. In *Philosophy of Ethics, Alterity and the Other*, ed. Ronald C. Arnett and Patricia Arneson, 87–106. Madison: Farleigh Dickinson University Press.

Manning, Erin. 2020. *For a Pragmatics of the Useless.* Durham: Duke University Press.

McCaffrey, Tony. 2023. *Giving and Taking Voice in Learning Disabled Theatre.* London: Routledge.

Savarese, David James. 2024. Mary Swander's Emerging Voices: The Only Neuro I Know. https://swander.substack.com/p/the-only-neuro-i-know Accessed 18th August 2024.

The Journeyings of Different Light. 2022. Devised by Different Light Theatre. Directed by Tony McCaffrey. ADSA Conference, University of Auckland, 6–9 Dec.

CHAPTER 3

Southside Stories: Pacific Artists, Funding, Evaluation and Wellbeing in South Auckland

Michelle Johansson

Ngā Mihi

Kei aku nui, kei aku rahi, kua hui mai nei ki raro i te mana o te whare e tū nei, tēnā koutou katoa.

This chapter begins in Te Reo Māori, the Indigenous language of Aotearoa New Zealand, offering thanks and greetings to the readers, and acknowledging the volume that houses this work. Firmly rooted in the creative tūāpapa (foundation) of South Auckland, this is an exploration of the impact of policy, funding and evaluation in the Arts and in Education on the young artists and activists of my community. Beginning with a close look at the work of the Black Friars theatre company project *Southside Rise,* attention will be drawn to the danger of policy-making and the associated funding mechanisms and evaluation systems that are designed "about us and without us". Like young activist Calista Fa'amausili, cited

M. Johansson (✉)
Ako Mātātupu: Teach First NZ, Auckland, New Zealand
e-mail: michelle.johansson@teachfirstnz.org

M. Mullen et al. (eds.), *Artful Evaluation for Creative Health and Wellbeing*, New Directions in Cultural Policy Research,
https://doi.org/10.1007/978-3-032-17063-7_3

later in this chapter, I hope that one day, communities like mine will function with self-determination and equal access to resources that will secure their powerful participation in the Arts and its associated benefits, including strong cultural identity and holistic wellbeing (Fig. 3.1).

Southside Rise is a movement begun in 2017 as a collaboration between my theatre company, the Black Friars, and 14 secondary schools serving low-income communities in South Auckland, Aotearoa New Zealand. In 2017, the Black Friars invited young activists and artists to come and tell their own stories of South Auckland through theatre (Tapaleao 2017). *Southside Rise* was the first production of its kind and, through performance, we worked to build a village that would challenge predominant national narratives about literacy, leadership and perceptions of South Auckland (Moimoiseā 2019). Over three years, we worked with over 100 young people to produce three full-scale original theatre shows with a full band and original music and dance. We were able to reach over 4,000 audience members from the community and beyond. The

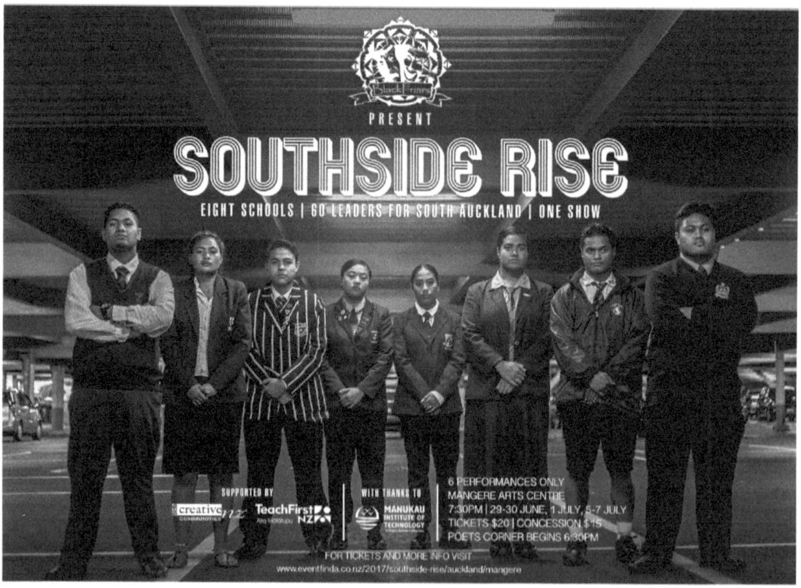

Fig. 3.1 *Southside Rise* poster, by L. Folau and F. Fifita (2017). Reprinted with permission

participants involved in the *Southside Rise* productions have continued to work with us, perform with us and walk beside us. They have become council members, climate change warriors, parents, nurses, journalists and teachers. They have signed modelling contracts, joined acting agencies and represented Aotearoa in international festivals. Many of them formed deep connections and lasting relationships through *Southside Rise.* Most of them have enduring and close contact with at least one of the older Black Friars. These Pasifika change-makers are steeped in what Karlo Mila terms "Polycultural capital" (Mila-Schaaf and Robinson 2010). Polycultural capital "describes the potential advantage Pacific second generation (New Zealand-born) may experience from ongoing exposure to culturally distinctive social spaces" (Mila-Schaaf and Robinson 2010, 1). Mila-Schaaf (2010, 1) argues that "having Pacific cultural capital as well as capital sourced to dominant social spaces assists in realising cumulative advantage and may be associated with improved education outcomes". For our *Southside Rise* participants, Polycultural capital meant actively and consciously honing the strengths and skills needed for Indigenous people to walk tall in two worlds—the first being the Western, colonial, world whose systems govern most elements of our everyday lives in Aotearoa, New Zealand; and the other being the Pasifika worlds that they, their families and communities inhabit. Now in their mid-twenties, *Southside Rise* alumni speak confidently to the ways in which their collective experience of the project contributed to their life-long understandings of hauora (holistic wellbeing), identity and culture.

This chapter is focused on the past, present and future impact of policy, funding and evaluation on those 150-plus young, brown scholars who are part of the *Southside Rise* movement. Policy and evaluation are intrinsically connected. Policy defines what is valued by our nation, and evaluation determines how we measure or 'count' it. With this framing in mind, *Southside Rise* was designed to grow leaders for South Auckland, steeped in Indigenous Pacific literacies and equipped to make change in their communities. Six years since the project's inception, and invested in the understanding "that solutions to problems already exist within communities, and the aim is to identify potentially transferable behaviours and enabling factors that are useful" (Mila-Schaaf 2013, 30), the young warriors of Southside Rise still proclaim vehemently that "only the hood, can heal the hood". In terms of value and valuation, it is important to reflect on what is counted by government funding initiatives and what 'counts' in the life trajectories of our young people.

The *Southside Rise* village created by and with these young people has been a powerful way of nurturing a collective identity, developing shared awareness of social injustice and galvanising action in the community—all facets of strong Polycultural capital. One young leader remarks that:

> No matter how hard I tried as a student I thought the problem was me. It was as if I had to constantly apologize for coming from a low socioeconomic background or from South Auckland. Now I embrace my successes and being from the south because… I see that it is not our students that fail, it's the education system that's failing our students. (L. Anae, personal correspondence, 1 September, 2017)

Through the distance-framing of performance, the young people were able to "speak openly about [their] cultures, [their] identities, about race and racism, gender bias, privilege and power", of how they underwent the "'un-learning' of ideas we never knew we held", and of their growing courage and conviction to stand up and be "brave warriors for social change" (Alesana, Folau, Milford, and Robertson-Johansson 2022, 117–8). In 2018, one of the wayfinders (young leaders) of this project wrote:

> I was asked what I hope for South Auckland…
>
> I hope that one day people realise
> we aren't just window washers and criminals
> but a place full of deadline meeters and high achievers.
> Communities full of tradition and hope.
> And this is where it all begins.
> This is how Southside will rise.
>
> Calista Fa'amausili, 17 years old – Tangaroa College Wayfinder
> *Southside Rise: Heads Held High, 2018.* (C. Fa'amausili, personal correspondence, 3 February; 2018)

For Calista and her peers, developing the collective Polycultural capital and agency of the village was paramount. However, despite the powerful affirmations of our young people, existing policies determine a very different approach to defining problems and what the successful, valued 'solutions' to those problems look like. The implicit 'value' embedded in policy and evaluation fail to support Mila-Schaaf's argument or the aspirations and experiences of the young warriors of Southside Rise.

Pasifika Positionality in Aotearoa New Zealand

Pacific Peoples constitute an estimated nine per cent of the population of Aotearoa New Zealand.[1] We are *tagata o le moana* (people of the ocean), closely related—culturally, genealogically, socio-economically and geographically—to tangata whenua (people of the land - Māori). While we are not indigenous to Aotearoa, we are nonetheless linked by blood ties and diasporic indigeneity to our Māori kin. Moreover, the colonial government of Aotearoa frequently connects Māori and Pacific Peoples through policies, initiatives, strategies and schemes to address our collective underrepresentation in positive outcomes (education, income, home ownership) and our overrepresentation in negative outcomes (incarceration, widespread underachievement, ill-health). In this chapter, I also use the term 'Pasifika'. Despite the fact that this term was initially introduced as a way to systematically group the many disparate Pacific migrants to Aotearoa New Zealand and is often statistically weaponised, 'Pasifika' nonetheless feels like a word of the Pacific. Using this term, in this context, is a reclamation of a collective identity, rather than an acquiescence to colonial efforts to homogenise the many diverse peoples of Oceania who call Aotearoa home.

I am an Aotearoa-born Pasifika theatre-maker and educator, working in the contested spaces of the performing arts and education where theory meets practice, in the heart of South Auckland. For my mother, emigrating from the small island of Tonga in the 1970s, Aotearoa was the proverbial 'land of milk and honey'. This vision of Aotearoa, as seen from the smaller Pacific Islands, obscured the complicated relationship between Mana Whenua (those with indigenous, territorial rights over tribal land) and Tauiwi (foreigners, visitors, non-Māori) and consequently discouraged connections between Pasifika immigrants and their Māori kin. The colonial government thus created an enduring divide between peoples who should have been each other's closest allies.

There are a myriad of policies targeted at Pasifika youth in Aotearoa, issued by the many arms of New Zealand's colonial government. From

[1] https://www.stats.govt.nz/topics/population/.

the Ministry for Pacific Peoples, where "Pacific communities are recognised for the diversity they bring, the knowledge they impart and the contribution they make to the uniqueness of Aotearoa" (Sio 2018, 5), to Auckland Council, who promise to "celebrate [their] uniqueness and achievements" (Auckland Council 2020, 23). However, beyond these broad, sweeping public statements, there is also an understanding that "in New Zealand socio-economic disadvantage has a large overlap with ethnicity … which affects Māori and Pacific students disproportionately" (The Southern Initiative 2020, 17) and that there continue to be "disparities in access to education and health services for Māori and Pacific children and their families; and [a] disproportionate number of Māori and Pacific People in poverty and material hardship" (New Zealand Government 2019, 12). This double-messaging promotes the overall perception that while Aotearoa loves her Pacific Peoples and their cultures, is proud of them and wants them to do well, for some (mysterious) reason, they keep popping up at the bottom end of all the statistics. On the one hand, government policies might be understood as the benevolent practice of addressing the problem of an inherently inferior Pacific population. On the other hand, government policies might be better understood as the patronising practice of maintaining power and dominance over a growing portion of the population that it deliberately, consistently and systematically fails in each and every way.

For Pasifika young people living in South Auckland, this systemic failure is exacerbated by geography and demographics. While they live in Auckland, the "first city of the Pacific" (Auckland Council 2018, 19), their locale is marked by extreme poverty, overcrowding, ill-health, crime, transience and media representations that position them as both dangerous and endangered (New Zealand Government 2019, 12). Policy paints these young people as the nation's 'at risk' 'priority learners'. And yet, young leaders, like Calista (quoted above), do not see themselves as pitiable or inferior. Instead, they require government policy, funding and evaluation systems that value Pasifika strengths, rather than policy that patronises their people, while measuring their individual and collective worth solely by their proximity to whiteness.

Policy History and Context

The colonial government of New Zealand has made the 'long brown tail of underachievement' (in Education, Employment, Income, Health, Housing and Wellbeing) one of the "problematizations through which we are governed" (Bacchi 2012, 4). Problematising Pacific Peoples through policies designed to "fix" the deficits in their cultural identity has been the pattern in government strategies over the last 20 years (Si'ilata, Samu and Siteine 2017, 6; Mullen and Johansson 2020), and while strengths-based change has been signalled—including change rooted in Polycultural capital—this is yet to be realised in lived experience.

Historically, government support for the arts began in the 1940s, when the Ministry of Cultural Affairs (now Manatū Taonga | the Ministry of Culture and Heritage) was established. In 2024, Manatū Taonga outlines their purpose as delivering on the "Government's priorities of improving the quality of public spending and regulation, lifting New Zealand's productivity and economic growth and increasing opportunities and prosperity for all New Zealanders", further cautioning that "in the current fiscal environment, we need to be more deliberate about how we use government funding" (Manatū Taonga | Ministry for Culture and Heritage 2024, 4).

The Arts Council of New Zealand Toi Aotearoa Act 2014 includes a mandate to recognise and uphold the principles of participation, access, excellence, professionalism and advocacy, and Pacific Peoples are named in Part 1, Sect. 3.3 (1)(c): "recognise the arts of the Pacific Island peoples of New Zealand" (Arts Council of New Zealand Toi Aotearoa Act 2014). These clauses are unchanged from the 1994 version of the Act. Creative New Zealand, the operational arm of the Arts Council with the responsibility for determining funding, building capability and international relations, created a process and timeline for reviewing its support for Pacific arts (Creative NZ 2013). The Creative New Zealand Pacific Arts sector consultation and review 2013, and the Arts Council of New Zealand Toi Aotearoa Act 2014 were integral to the direction setting for the current Pacific Arts Strategy 2023–2028 and accompanying document, the Investment Strategy Te Ara Whakamua 2018–2023.

The 2013 review importantly found that a greater allocation of funding was needed for Pacific arts and Pasifika artists, and specific areas for increased support and improvement of understanding were identified as part of the strategic plan for the next five years (Creative NZ 2013, 3).

Included in this review are reflections from Pacific artists who express a lack of confidence in the Arts Council. Significantly, these reflections indicate a mismatch between Creative NZ's existing systems and processes, and the Pacific artists they are meant to serve. One said, "CNZ's whole approach needs to be re-looked at as it is not working. More money needs to go into going out to these [heritage arts] communities and working with them instead of trying to get them to come to you with a huge English document that straight away puts up a huge block" (Creative NZ 2013). By the time of the Pacific Arts Strategy 2023–2028, the shift in the Arts Council to support Pacific Peoples to be self-determining is emphasised in the five-year strategic direction for "a longer-term sustainable impact on people, communities and ecosystems" (Creative NZ 2023a, 8). The 2023 Pacific Arts Strategy is a stake in the ground for Pacific arts and artists. Founded on Indigenous Pacific concepts—Tagata, Vaka, Va and Moana[2]—the strategy encompasses investment, development, leadership, advocacy, encouragement, promotion and support for the arts and artists of the Pacific. Similarly, the Investment Plan includes a mandate to "actively work to increase Creative New Zealand's capacity and capability around Pacific arts, to ensure the success of this Strategy", including recruiting more Pasifika staff (Creative NZ 2019, 9). The principles that underpin the Pacific Arts Strategy are manifested in the actions of the Investment Plan and supported by a commitment to employ Pasifika staff as cultural experts to grow the understanding of the entire organisation.

In early November 2024, Amplify: A Creative and Cultural Strategy for New Zealand (draft), was launched. Amplify outlines how the government will prioritise support for our creative and cultural sectors to 2030, setting out how existing levels of funding will be used "for maximum impact, purposefully leveraging further investment from other actors" (Goldsmith 2024, 3). Among its intentions, Amplify pledges that the government will collaborate across the creative sector "to make existing funding channels easier to access and navigate, promote and supplement other revenue channels, and explore new opportunities for cultural practitioners to earn income" (Manatū Taonga | Ministry for Culture &

[2] Tagata = people; Vaka = the boat, or vessel, which signifies the great ocean-going traditions of the Pacific; Va = the relational spaces that connect us; Moana = the Pacific Ocean. These are all easily identified symbols of the lived experience and ways of being of Pacific Peoples.

Heritage 2024, 16). While the aspiration to make funding more accessible to arts practitioners is admirable, Amplify also places much emphasis on the economic value of the arts to Aotearoa and the potential of creative and cultural products for export. The strategy expresses the importance of opportunities to "take advantage of a growing digital export market, reach new audiences, create innovative products, and support social outcomes" and goes on to highlight that "global measures of soft power indicate that New Zealand's international reputation for business and trade is an advantage that can be leveraged" (Manatū Taonga | Ministry for Culture & Heritage 2024, 16). The strategy is clear that the government will remain within "current levels of funding" for the arts, but that practitioners should also consider the value of those same arts as commodities to be sold for financial gain. Projects like *Southside Rise* are unlikely to fall into the governmental priorities of creative arts ready for export and it is of concern that Amplify focuses on the economic importance of the arts and largely overlooks the enormous benefits of the creative arts to the collective social and cultural good. For companies like mine, working with communities in building identity, culture and belonging through the arts, the ability to access funding will be severely limited at best and at worst, non-existent.

One of the most significant barriers to creating policy that serves Pacific Peoples is the failure of ministries to work strategically, systemically and connectedly. The Child and Youth Wellbeing Strategy, 2019—one of the only cross-government strategies—acknowledges the "fragmentation of effort" across departments and policies, saying that "at a public policy level there are too many policies that were developed and implemented in silos" (New Zealand Government 2019, 13). It is partly due to this fragmentation of effort that policies and strategies are created that do not work for Pacific Peoples *by design* (Duncan-Andrade 2017). Duncan-Andrade argues that colonial systems fail minority groups deliberately and strategically in order to maintain the dominance and power of the status quo. Policy amendments are then created to cater to the otherness of Pacific Peoples, and these amendments have significant impact. Firstly, and at best, they position Pacific Peoples as slightly remedial, not unlike the primitive islands from which they come. Secondly, these amendments typically either lower the bar for Pacific Peoples to 'catch up' to their white counterparts, or they are designed to berate individuals (such as teachers) for failing to make the system "fit" their Pacific clientele. The Action Plan for Pacific Education (APPE) may be considered one such amendment. The *APPE* leans into all three of these potential impacts by describing educational outcomes that might even be "within reach" of Pacific learners; by promising to alleviate "financial barriers to access" and the "affordability" of uniform and devices; and by mandating cultural responsiveness training for teachers (Ministry of Education 2020, 8–9). Viewed as a list, these actions might seem perfectly reasonable, but they are also indicators of a system that created the poverty and disadvantage in the first place.

Young Pasifika South Aucklanders are particularly susceptible victims of policy. Bacchi (2012, 4) argues that "we are all located within practices and problematizations that shape us to an extent, it is difficult to stand back and study their operation", and this is substantiated by Leah's statement that "no matter how hard I tried as a student I thought the problem was me" (personal correspondence, 1 September, 2017). Council documents admit that "the north–south motorway has become the divide between rich and poor… All the way around the Manukau Harbour there is a swathe of deprivation" (Auckland Council 2020, 21) and that "South Aucklanders were working more hours and getting paid less than other Aucklanders for many of the same types of jobs" (The Southern Initiative 2020, 59). However, there is no concerted, collective effort by either local or national government to address this inequality in a wholesale and systemic way. Instead, we live in a system where the young Pasifika boy growing up in poverty is clearly deserving of our pity, and yet, when the child that we pity grows into the man that we fear—we punish him for it.

Only the Hood can Heal the Hood

In *Southside Rise: Revolution*, six young people in a detention room discuss success in the school system:

TAI: But that's not how YOU fight. People respect your word, that's your power.
YOU win by speaking your truth.

MAIA: Truth? The truth is, we were never meant to succeed. Not like this. Not as.
ourselves. How can we? The game is rigged. We're done. I'm done.

TOA: Done? We haven't even started.

(From *Southside Rise: Revolution*. M. Alefosio, G. Faatau'uu-Satiu, I. B. Johansson, M. Johansson, V. Johansson, B. Revell-Sio, D. Su'a, T. Telea, R. Worley 2019).

Mullen et al. (2020, 2), working closely with the Black Friars, state that "historically, Pasifika young people have been represented in policy as vulnerable, struggling, at risk of poor social outcomes and, as a result, in need of targeted corrective interventions". They go on to describe the need for strengths-based policy and self-determination. Even Auckland Council understands that "in Aotearoa a strengths-based approach and meaningful cultural intelligence applied at a local level is fundamental to address the inherent racism, bias and low expectations for Māori and Pasifika ākonga in the mainstream system" (The Southern Initiative 2020, 20). However, 'strengths-based' is currently an objective term that is not well understood by governing authorities, and Polycultural capital, even less so.

In 2023, *New Zealanders and the Arts Ko Aotearoa me ōna Toi* was published, highlighting the important connections between the arts and wellbeing. Based on the 7000 + responses, there is a significant upward trend in the number of New Zealanders who appreciate the difference the arts make to social and collective wellbeing. The survey notes that 63% of respondents claim that the arts are good for their mental health and wellbeing and 68% note that they learn about different cultures through the arts (Creative NZ 2023b, 5–6). The study also shows that participation and attendance in the arts have risen across all parts of society and that young people, deaf and disabled, Māori and Pacific peoples participate in the arts most frequently (Creative NZ 2023b, 15). The report suggests strong links between the arts and wellbeing, which resonate with the vitality of the Southside Rise village.

Our young performers told us that:

> Theatre saves lives. And the village we've built through the theatre continues to save lives... There are bonds created in the theatre that turn into lifelong friendships, and into lifelines in times of crisis. There have been times over the last five years of this work that each of us has been desperate, depressed or lost, and the bonds we built through theatre have been the thing that has pulled us back. We've made the 3am calls to each other to check in and to reach out. Our understanding of the theatre is

> that because it has created a space where we have been vulnerable together, this means that we will never have to be vulnerable alone. (Alesana et al. 2022, 118)

While *Amplify* does at least acknowledge that "creative and cultural activity does not only benefit the cultural sector. There are wider benefits delivered across sectors, including economic, social and wellbeing benefits" (Manatū Taonga | Ministry for Culture & Heritage 2024, 17), a deeper understanding of these "wellbeing benefits" is needed, particularly what wellbeing benefits might mean to Pacific youth, as well as a way to reflect these benefits in funding allocation. Aotearoa needs a society-wide awareness and appreciation of the arts and the enormous role they have in fostering collective wellbeing and social cohesion. These are the elements that the Southside Rise young people value and that continue to form those 'lifelines in times of crisis' that are needed more and more among all young people in Aotearoa.

There are a wide range of policies that have and continue to affect the young Pasifika people involved in *Southside Rise,* from policy and strategy documents focused on the Pacific Arts and their exportability and potential financial value, as well as a plethora of Pacific Education policies that position them as liabilities, in need of remedial assistance. None of these policies value or acknowledge the Polycultural capital wielded by these young people every day, or are able to measure the immense social and cultural benefits of participating in the creative arts. The upward swing in life trajectories of the alumni of the *Southside Rise* movement illustrates how the creative arts can meaningfully and irrevocably improve lives; however, these are not the outcomes that are measured or 'counted' in current policy in Aotearoa.

Funding

Centralised government funding for the arts is administered by Creative NZ. Each of their large Arts Grants includes the option to be considered specifically under Pacific criteria, and there are grants under the Pasifika Festivals Initiative of up to $150,000, as well as the Creative NZ Arts Pasifika Awards which recognise the achievement of individual artists. The Creative Communities Scheme consists of small allocations of funding (under $2,000) which are administered by local government.

In the last Arts Grants funding round, four projects in the Pacific Arts, totalling $250,000, were supported (Creative NZ 2024).

Despite these efforts by Creative NZ, funding remains the most significant challenge and threat to Pasifika artists. Recent funding initiatives, for example, are designed to support individual or small groups of practitioners, rather than the villages that are formed in creating works such as *Southside Rise*. There is little to no consideration from Creative NZ for large casts and crew, which are difficult to sustain financially (Johansson 2023). A simple example of the mismatch between what is considered of worth to fund by CNZ and what Pacific artists need and value is the fact that Creative NZ will not sponsor food for a company, which is a fundamental connector for Pacific Peoples.

The Diversity in the Arts Policy determines that Creative NZ (2015, 2) "will ensure there are no significant barriers to accessing our support and our resources". However, while efforts to provide targeted funding for the Pacific Arts have improved, the actual frameworks for funding mentioned in the 2013 review remain entrenched in colonial ways of being. These include long application forms, dense English language and the requirement for artists to be registered legal entities to access the larger funds. This requirement carries with it ongoing economic implications which fail to reflect the collective or temporal nature of Pacific arts-making.

Data Sources

The Organisation for Economic Co-operation and Development (OECD) (2012) describes the governance of Aotearoa's education system as "shared between the central government and schools", and this dichotomy seems indicative of government policy more generally. Legislation, policy and strategy documents, as well as funding applications and information on those who receive funding are publicly available and easy to access. However, there is a significant gap between the high-level vision of the government and how that vision makes its way to the people on the ground. The statement by the OECD emphasises the fact that while centralised government policies are aspirational, the process by which these aspirations are grounded in schools, or local bodies, is inconsistent, systemically biased, and ultimately flawed. An example of this might be seen in the work of Stats NZ, which reports census data but cannot, by design, serve those who are disenfranchised and mistrusting of the government (e.g. Aotearoa's 40,000 + rough sleepers—Amore 2016) and are consequently 'not counted' in future government planning.

This idea of 'not being counted' is further exacerbated by research conducted by the government, whose primary means of 'consultation' is by online survey (e.g. Creative NZ, 2013). Research, by these means, is anti-Indigenous, deeply suspicious and frequently harmful. As Kukutai and Cormack (2020, 22) argue:

> The approach to Indigenous policy has long been to contain and manage, rather than to enable genuine forms of Indigenous self-determination or autonomy. To give full effect to IDS—that is, for Indigenous Peoples to determine the means of collection, access, analysis, interpretation, management, dissemination and reuse of data from or pertaining to them requires a level of Indigenous power and autonomy within State systems that does not currently exist.

Thus, Pasifika people, who are already disadvantaged by colonial systems, become further 'other'-ised in the surveying of those same systems and do not or cannot engage with the evaluation of what data is collected and how well it represents and serves them.

Community and Industry

There are many groups serving South Auckland in the spaces of Activism, Education and the Arts and there is a substantial and growing number of community-led, grass-roots organisations taking action in South Auckland—for Pasifika, by Pasifika. From adult-led community groups such as Siaola (founded 2018), Affirming Works (founded 2001), Pasefika Proud (founded 2008), Ura Tabu (founded 2012) and Grow Boundary (founded 2021); through to more recent youth-led groups, such as 4TK - 4 Tha Kulture (founded 2019), Do Good Feel Good (founded 2017), Brown Pride (founded 2020), UMU (founded 2020) and Tu Fa'atasi (founded 2020). Specially engaged in the work of reclaiming the Southside story through the arts are Odd Family (founded 2019), Black Friars (founded 2006), Sau e Siva (founded 2016), Brave (founded 2021) and MMØS (founded 2017).

While this rising village of activists and artists is enormously positive, the current structure of accessible funding necessarily puts them in competition with each other, rather than allowing for a linking of hands across the sector. The competitive nature of contestable funding engenders unnecessary animosity between organisations who are composed of and serve the same people. Once again, colonial structures have created a divide between Pacific Peoples.

Recommendations

This chapter concludes with three recommendations for policy design that have the potential to effect change with and for young brown scholars on the Southside. Firstly, immediate and cohesive work is needed by government on both self-awareness and understanding multiple worldviews from indigenous perspectives. In Education and the Arts, this means starting with existing scholarship. Tongan scholar, Karlo Mila-Schaaf (2010), coined the term 'Polycultural capital' to describe the unique strengths, skills and knowledges that are held by Pacific People, and Si'ilata et al. (2017) offer the Va'a Tele—the Samoan double-hulled canoe as a tangible and clear means of understanding the two worlds in which Pacific learners must function. Leaning on the existing frameworks presented by indigenous leaders will help to grow a collective national understanding of Pacific strengths.

Secondly, there are vital links between the arts, culture and wellbeing that are undervalued and not well understood by government agencies. Despite the fact that much emerging research, as well as the government's own reports, points to the direct correlation between the arts and mental health and wellbeing, there is little evidence of increased investment in this medicine that we know works. While the mental health of Aotearoa is in crisis and our suicide rate still ranks among the highest in the developed world (Te Whatu Ora 2024), it is vital that we invest in our collective wellbeing in the ways that our young people are crying out for.

Finally, there will need to be long-term, strategic shift in government ways of working. This includes holistic system change; a repositioning of legislation, policy and strategy based on multiple world views; and a nationwide commitment to governance that serves Māori first. Any policy that requires a targeted corrective intervention for Māori or Pacific Peoples must be called out as racist. If this is understood well and undertaken without resentment or ego, then it will no longer be necessary for Pacific People "to clothe themselves with the accoutrements of the dominant culture, in order to be seen to be successful in their migrant home" (Si'ilata et al. 2017, 26). There is a commitment made in the opening lines of the *APPE*, that the government will work to "transform our education system to better serve our Pacific learners" (Ministry of Education 2018, 5). However, this society-wide transformation cannot occur "without us and about us" for the young Pacific warriors of South Auckland. Meaningful change is only possible if the "essential partnerships" (4) promised in the *APPE* are also equal.

Conclusion

There are many representations of Aotearoa New Zealand as a multicultural utopia—clean, green and fair. We have a world-class education system, a stable economy and an accommodating climate year-round. However, this vision of the country conceals its complicated history and privileges "the power holders without appearing to claim any privilege" (Greenwood and Wilson 2006, 85). In the arts and education sectors, policy has been used to promote public perception of a benevolent government, engaged in remedial efforts to help its Māori and Pacific subjects, who are backward by nature.

Pasifika youth on the Southside have long been governed by a system deliberately designed to ensure their failure. While local government prides itself on being "the first city of the Pacific [with] the greatest number of Pacific residents on the planet" (Auckland Council 2018, 19), those same governing bodies have yet to realise the full potential of their young, brown warriors. Problematising policy, evaluation and funding from a Pacific perspective necessarily means understanding that all policies and strategies designed to 'save' Pacific young people from themselves would be immediately redundant if governing systems served their people as equal and essential partners.

References

Alesana, Patrick., Irene Folau, Agnes Milford, Linda Robertson-Johansson. 2022. Theatre to Raise a Village. In *The Routledge companion to theatre and young people*, eds. Selina Busby, Kelly Freebody, and Charlene Rajendran, 117–118. London: Routledge.

Amore, Kate. 2016. Severe housing deprivation in Aotearoa/New Zealand: 2001–2013. He Kainga Oranga/Housing & Health Research Programme, University of Otago, Wellington. https://www.healthyhousing.org.nz/sites/default/files/2024-05/Severe%20housing%20deprivation%20in%20Aotearoa%202001-2013_0.pdf. Accessed 8 July 2025

Arts Council of New Zealand Toi Aotearoa Act. 2014. https://www.legislation.govt.nz/act/public/2014/0001/latest/whole.html?search=ta_act%40act_A_ac%40ainf%40anif%40aaif_ac%40bn%40rn_25_a&p=6#DLM3007315. Accessed 8 July 2025

Auckland Council. 2020. Te Mahere Ā-Rohe O Māngere-Ōtāhuhu 2020: Māngere-Ōtāhuhu Local Board Plan 2020. Auckland Council. https://www.aucklandcouncil.govt.nz/about-auckland-council/how-auckland-council-works/local-boards/all-local-boards/mangere-otahuhu-local-board/Documents/mangere-otahuhu-local-board-plan-english-2020.pdf. Accessed 8 July 2025

Auckland Council. 2018. Auckland Plan 2050. Auckland Council. https://www.aucklandcouncil.govt.nz/plans-projects-policies-reports-bylaws/our-plans-strategies/auckland-plan/Pages/default.aspx. Accessed 8 July 2025

Bacchi, Carol. 2012. Why study problematizations? Making politics visible. *Open Journal of Political Science* 2. no. 01: 1–8

Creative NZ. 2013. Creative New Zealand Pacific Arts sector consultation and review 2013. Creative NZ: Arts Council of New Zealand Toi Aotearoa.

Creative NZ. 2015. Diversity in the Arts Policy, October 2015. Creative NZ: Arts Council of New Zealand Toi Aotearoa.

Creative NZ. 2019. Pacific Arts Strategy 2018–2023—Implementation Plan. Creative NZ: Arts Council of New Zealand Toi Aotearoa.

Creative NZ. 2023a. Pacific Arts Strategy 2023–2028. Creative NZ: Arts Council of New Zealand Toi Aotearoa. https://creativenz.govt.nz/-/media/project/creative-nz/creativenz/publicationsfiles/2023-pacific-arts-strategy/2023-pacific-strategy_final.pdf. Accessed 8 May 2025

Creative NZ. 2023b. New Zealanders and the Arts Ko Aotearoa me ōna Toi. Creative NZ: Arts Council of New Zealand Toi Aotearoa. https://creativenz.govt.nz/-/media/project/creative-nz/creativenz/publicationsfiles/2024-nzers-and-the-arts/20240417-summaryreport-final.pdf. Accessed 8 May 2025.

Creative NZ. 2024. Creative Impact Fund 2024 - Round 1. Creative NZ: Arts Council of New Zealand Toi Aotearoa. https://creativenz.govt.nz/funding-and-support/results/funding-rounds/creative-impact-fund-2024---round-1. Accessed 8 May 2025

Duncan-Andrade, Jeff. 2017. The game is rigged (inequity by design). Teach For All. https://vimeo.com/234442724. Accessed 8 May 2025.

Goldsmith, Paul. 2024. Minister's Foreword. In *Amplify: A creative and cultural strategy for New Zealand (draft)*. Wellington: Manatū Taonga | Ministry of Culture and Heritage. https://www.mch.govt.nz/sites/default/files/2024-11/amplify%E2%80%93creative_and_cultural_strategy_for_new_zealand_2024%E2%80%932030_0.pdf. Accessed 8 May 2025.

Greenwood, Janinka, and A. Wilson. 2006. Stories whispered by the land: An account of two workshop events, in Parua Bay and Te Kaha. Canterbury University. https://ir.canterbury.ac.nz/server/api/core/bitstreams/37833d0a-ac2e-448d-9be8-cc39ddba2b43/content. Accessed 8 May 2025.
Johansson, Michelle. 2023. Theater, drama, education, and Pasifika youth in Aotearoa New Zealand. In *Oxford Research Encyclopedia of Education*. https://doi.org/10.1093/acrefore/9780190264093.013.1719. Accessed 8 July 2025.
Kukutai, Tahu, and Donna Cormack. 2020. "Pushing the space": Data sovereignty and self-determination in Aotearoa NZ. In *Indigenous data sovereignty and policy,* eds. Tahu Kukutai, Donna Cormack, Maggie Walter, Stephanie Russo Carroll, and Desi Rodriguez-Lonebear, 21–35. London: Routledge
Manatū Taonga | Ministry for Culture & Heritage. 2021. General directions of cultural policy. Cultural Policy in New Zealand. https://mch.govt.nz/cultural-policy-new-zealand/1-general-directions-cultural-policy. Accessed 8 May 2025.
Manatū Taonga | Ministry for Culture & Heritage. 2024. Amplify—A creative and cultural strategy for New Zealand (DRAFT—NOT GOVERNMENT POLICY). https://www.mch.govt.nz/sites/default/files/2024 11/amplify%E2%80%93creative_and_cultural_strategy_for_new_zealand_2024%E2%80%932030_0.pdf. Accessed 8 May 2025.
Mila-Schaaf, Karlo, and Elizabeth Robinson. 2010. Polycultural capital and educational achievement among NZ-born Pacific peoples. *Mai review* 1: 1–18.
Mila-Shaaf, Karlo. 2013. Not another New Zealand-born identity crisis: Well-being and the politics of belonging. In *Pacific identities and well-being: Cross-cultural perspectives*, eds. Agee, Margaret Nelson, Tracey McIntosh, Philip Culbertson, and Cabrini 'Ofa Makasiale, 27–45. London: Routledge
Ministry of Education. 2020. Action plan for Pacific education: 2020–2030. Ministry of Education. https://conversation.education.govt.nz/conversations/action-plan-for-pacific-education/. Accessed 8 May 2025
Ministry of Social Development. 2021. Request for proposals: Youth engagement programme. Ministry of Social Development. Auckland.
Momoiseā, Destiny. 2019. Southside Rise—Revolution. The Coconet. https://www.thecoconet.tv/coco-talanoa/events/southside-rise-revolution/. Accessed 8 May 2025.
Mullen, Molly. 2021. Holding it together: Resilience and solidarity in the economies of Auckland youth performance companies. *Research in Drama Education: The Journal of Applied Theatre and Performance* 26, no. 1: 88–104
Mullen, Molly, Amber Walls, Maria Ahmad, and Peter O'Connor. 2023. Resourcing the arts for youth wellbeing: Challenges in Aotearoa New Zealand. *Arts & Health* 15, no. 1: 71–85

Mullen, Molly, Michelle Johansson, Ashleigh Niuia, 'Iunisi Bayley Johansson, Billy Revell-Sīo, Carmel Maria Savaiinaea, Faananaafu Tofilau, Leonard Folau, Maria Ahmad and Viola Johansson. 2020. Opening doors, not filling boxes: Policy kinesis and youth performance with the Black Friars theatre company, Aotearoa New Zealand. In *The Applied Theatre Reader*, eds. Tim Prentki and Nicola Abraham, 278–285. London: Routledge

New Zealand Government. 2019. Child and youth wellbeing strategy. https://childyouthwellbeing.govt.nz/resources/child-and-youth-wellbeing-strategy-html. Accessed 8 May 2025.

Organisation for Economic Co-operation and Development. 2012. Education policy outlook snapshot: New Zealand. OECD Better policies for better lives. https://www.oecd.org/education/highlightsnewzealand.htm. Accessed 8 May 2025

Si'ilata, Rae., Tanya Wendt Samu, and Alexis Siteine. 2017. The va 'atele framework: Redefining and transforming Pasifika education. In *Handbook of indigenous education*, eds. Elizabeth Ann McKinley, and Linda Tuhiwai Smith, 1–30. Springer

Sio, S. W., 2018. Pacific Aotearoa Lalanga Fou. Ministry for Pacific Peoples. https://www.mpp.govt.nz/assets/Reports/Pacific-Aotearoa-Lalanga-Fou-Report.pdf. Accessed 8 May 2025.

Tapaleao, Vaimoana. 2017. *South Auckland student leaders unite for new production*. The New Zealand Herald, April 2017. https://www.nzherald.co.nz/nz/south-auckland-student-leaders-unite-for-new-production/VTB5LLC5RFMZ65LRAW7TSMMEIY/. Accessed 8 May 2025.

Te Whatu Ora. 2024. Suicide data web tool—Health New Zealand | Te Whatu Ora. Health New Zealand. https://www.tewhatuora.govt.nz/for-health-professionals/data-and-statistics/suicide/data-web-tool#:~:text=Overview,%2C%2012.1)%20per%20100%2C000%20population. Accessed 8 May 2024.

The Southern Initiative. 2020. Know me. Believe in me. Kia mārama mai, kia whakapono mai. Report by the Ministry of Education & The Southern Initiative. https://knowledgeauckland.org.nz/publications/know-me-believe-in-me-kia-marama-mai-kia-whakapono-mai/. Accessed 8 May 2025.

PART II

Justice-Oriented Evaluation

CHAPTER 4

Queevaluing The Coming Back Out Ball: Towards a Creative Framework of Self-Determined Values

Peta Murray, Marnie Badham, Tristan Meecham, and Bec Reid

Introduction

In this chapter, we draw upon discourses including queer theory, gerontology, and ritual studies to reflect on nuances of their engagement with All The Queens Men. We speak to the value of intergenerational, intersectional, and intercultural creative practices—and a need to re-imagine

P. Murray (✉) · M. Badham
RMIT University, Melbourne, VIC, Australia
e-mail: peta.murray2@rmit.edu.au

M. Badham
e-mail: marnie.badham@rmit.edu.au

T. Meecham · B. Reid
All the Queens Men, Melbourne, VIC, Australia
e-mail: tristan@allthequeensmen.net

B. Reid
e-mail: bec@allthequeensmen.net

M. Mullen et al. (eds.), *Artful Evaluation for Creative Health and Wellbeing*, New Directions in Cultural Policy Research,
https://doi.org/10.1007/978-3-032-17063-7_4

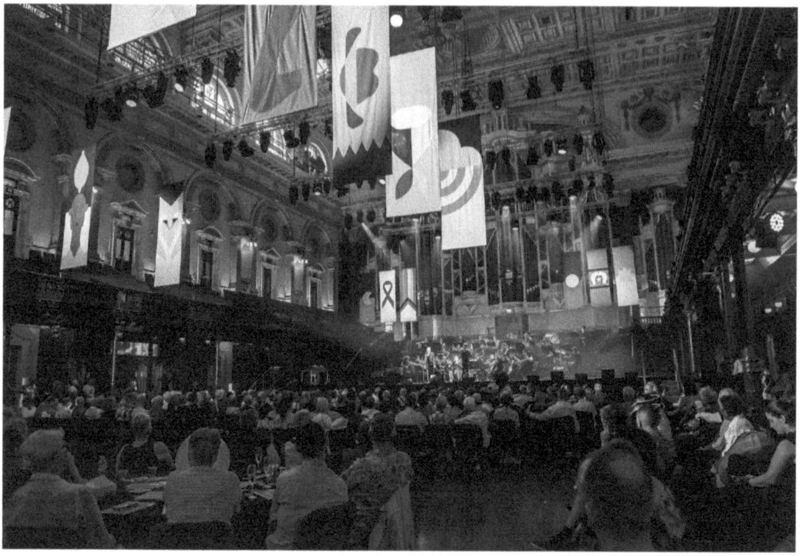

Fig. 4.1 The coming back out salon by All The Queens Men for Sydney World Pride. Image by Bryony Jackson (2023)

and self-determine approaches to evaluation as means to understand the significance of performance as a tool for care. Beyond interventions to address loneliness through building social connection and beyond celebrating queer and ageing identities, All The Queens Men continues to refine open-ended and innovative approaches we propose herein as *queevaluation* (Fig. 4.1).

Part One: In which We Map the Rainbow-Coloured Trail of the Coming Back Out Ball and the LGBTIQ+ Elders Dance Club across Australia

To the LGBTIQ+ elders who have led the way, who have shaped our communities, who have fought for our rights, we thank you. To the LGBTIQ+ elders who struggle to live their true sexual, gendered or cultural variation(s) because they don't feel safe, we are here for you. We

> offer this event to you as a gift; a gift in appreciation for all that you have done and with respect for all you have experienced.... The Coming Back Out Ball makes the invisible visible, the forgotten remembered, the past treasured and the present valued.

These words were offered in a toast to the community of LGBTIQ+ elders by Tristan Meecham, Artistic Director of independent Australian arts organisation All The Queen's Men in opening the inaugural Coming Back Out Ball as a premiere event of the 2017 Seniors Festival in Melbourne, Australia. As a young queer man, Tristan looked to those who had come before him and was moved to honour their stories through this spectacular event.

The Coming Back Out Ball was promoted as a once-in-a-lifetime event to celebrate the contributions and diversity of LGBTIQ+ elders. It was intended to combat loneliness and stigmatisation through opportunities for social bonding, connection to community, and by inviting culturally specific expressions of identity through dance and fashion (Badham et al. 2017). Born out of a social history of queer performance culture, The Coming Back Out Ball, an extravagant multi-arts spectacular, also nodded to traditions of gala Melbourne Balls of the 1970s and 1980s—key political and social activities for groups in the LGBTIQ+ community back in the day.

The timing was exquisite—and highly charged. Through 2016 and into 2017, several state governments in Australia offered formal apology and expungement of the criminal records of gay men for the *abominable crime of buggery* (Albion and Russell 2022; Boucher and Reynolds 2018). These coincided with the Australian government's *Same Sex Marriage Postal Vote* preparations. The delivery of these campaigns made the lives of LGBTIQ+ people a living hell, via a maelstrom of public debate and media stereotyping amid a frenzy of confected outrage and social division. Alongside this, emerging research on ageing in the LGBTIQ+ community identified a scourge of social isolation that was even more dangerous within elderly populations (Karp 2022; Barrett et al. 2025), particularly for those forced to live secretive lives due to bigotry and threats to their social and physical safety under state-sanctioned criminalisation and medicalisation protocols.

While marriage equality would be *granted*, no *Same Sex Marriage* referendum could expunge long held feelings of shame, erase stigma, or redress ostracism by family, friends, professional contexts, or community.

So, it was not surprising that research revealed many LGBTIQ+ elders were continuing to head *back into the closet* when they arrived at a stage of life where they sought access to aged care services and support (Barrett et al. 2025).

Such dispiriting research findings within increasingly complex cultural moments were the impetus for All The Queens Men to develop and deliver The Coming Back Out Ball. Melbourne-based allies from the community converged in response to All The Queens Men's call for volunteers, organisational partners, and an audience to bear witness to this historic event. An expansive media campaign profiled carefully nuanced representations of LGBTIQ+ elders and their stories (Joosten 2017), extending the message and its community-building initiative far and wide. As a glittering gala and gift to the community, The Coming Back Out Ball was received as a performed action full of meaning, feeling, connection, and intention. Meanwhile, as a launch, The Coming Back Out Ball positioned All The Queens Men among Australia's leading socially engaged performance art organisations. It soon gave rise to a suite of social Dance Club initiatives, delivered in person at local town halls and online during COVID-19 stay-at-home public health measures, to create communal events and experiences and hold space for LGBTIQ+ older people around the country. All The Queens Men has hosted these LGBTIQ+ Elders Dance Club events in Melbourne, Brisbane, Adelaide, Canberra, Sydney, Hobart, and throughout regional Victoria. Its core business continues to be giving *to*, giving *back*, giving *out*, and other kinds of prepositionally inflected interchange. Almost a decade on, All The Queens Men continues to curate events and community programmes specifically for LGBTIQ+ elders and their chosen families, friends, allies, and health providers. Recently, a new work, Play Date, has been devised and delivered for their children, grandchildren, niblings, and great niblings.

Part Two: In Which We *Out* Ourselves and Establish *Gifting* as a Metaphor of Significance

Core to our theorisation in this chapter are two concepts from the fields of anthropology and ritual studies, notably *communitas* and *the gift*. Communitas is understood as the spirit of community or as a common shared experience through rite of passage. In *Communitas: The*

Anthropology of Collective Joy, Edith Turner affords us a way to speak of experiences of liminality in which this unfettered joy may be transmuted and "*the gifts* of each and every person are alive to the fullest" (2012, 3, emphasis added). Of its value in research settings, Francesca Rendle-Short suggests that *communitas thinking* is a mode of practice that invites and gifts us "spaces and progressive structures and 'stories' of exchange and engagement that are non-acquisitional, ethical, mutually generative, and productive" (2021, 13). Marcel Mauss overturns transactional readings of the gift to identify generative networks of reciprocity (2002). If we posit communitas *as* gift, we may think of "togetherness itself" arising within cycles of mutuality and generosity in reciprocal exchange.

Through generous invitation, openness, and demonstration of integrity and obligation, All The Queens Men's aim for The Coming Back Out Ball was to celebrate and uplift LGBTIQ+ elders. In so doing, we are offered counternarratives to ageism, homophobia, and transphobia. These gifts are made through public gestures—some grand and lavish, others small and intimate—of seeing, centring, and illuminating queer lives and personalities. Through acts of acknowledgement, rites of elevation, and associated formalities, the boldness and beauty of members of the alphabet communities—who have led the way—are made visible.

I sneaked a cheeky *we* into the paragraph above. As co-author of this chapter, I, Peta Murray, wear assorted wigs/heels/leathers and feathers and must colour myself RAINBOW, *out* myself now—and do something nifty with pronouns—as a Seniors-Card-carrying member of All The Queens Men's queer constituency. I also moonlight as an academic alongside Marnie Badham, a friend and collaborator with All The Queens Men. As an artist-researcher, Badham is interested in how to shift the cultural capital of her university position to amplify, to activate, and to share resources with artists and community.

In other settings, we might be viewed as researcher-outsiders conducting fieldwork into the *exotic* world of All The Queens Men from the vantage point of the academy, but this is far from the case. Rather, we are a louche coalition of *paracademics*—Murray's term for scholars who are happier working alongside community rather than within the academy (Murray and Magner 2022). Both are immersed in the "programme" of All The Queens Men activity as constituents and participants, and Murray took a step towards a more embedded view and relationship, accepting an invitation to join All The Queens Men board of governance.

With expertise in socially engaged arts as a creative form of justice and care, Murray and Badham seek methodological insights through ethical practices that illuminate knowledge that already exists in these settings, and resist imposing external and often inappropriate value and values frameworks on culturally distinct communities. In fact, we go further in resisting official notions of value itself, in favour of methods that preference multivalent articulations of meaning and significance.

Here, Murray and Badham collaborate with duo *artistes* manifesting as art-husband Bec Reid and art-wife Tristan Meecham, the co-founding Artistic Directors of All The Queens Men. As *paracademics*, we refuse to collect data or extract stories on All The Queens Men's behalf, but rather, via durational and embedded approaches, support the artistes to do so themselves. As well as sharing insights arising, this chapter functions as an opportunity for reflection and provocation on their/our combined and collected observations, sense making, and motives for collaborating in and on this work.

I, Peta, am an older person, and a *wannabe eventual queer elder* in my community; so much so I claim coinage of the word *elderflowering* to speak to my ambitions for a blooming and preposterous old age (Murray 2017). I came into my own L-word in the late 1970s in Australia, conveniently timing a Sydney-based coming out story with burgeoning Gay Rights and Women's Movements (Willett 2013; Arrow and Woollacott 2020) and the vibrant social activism of the 78ers—those valiant souls who risked arrest when they processed along Sydney's Oxford Street in 1978 in part-parade, part protest (Simic 2017). This seemed as good a moment as any to be a lesbian in Australia, until AIDS tore through the communities of our gay brothers, and we all—dykes, poofs, queers and queens alike—were galvanised by shared purpose in a frantic quest to re-imagine care, and find meaning in the face of public hostility and waves of fear and loathing the epidemic had unleashed (Fela 2018; Sendziuk 2003).

With a new millennium and new pharmaceutical protocols, things settled somewhat. Gender and identity politics troubled so-called societal norms (Connell 2019; Ahmed 2010), while trans-advocacy (Feinberg 2013) and alternative familial notions of kith and kin (Halberstam 2011; Bradway and Freeman 2022), of intersectionality (Massaquoi 2015; Moreton Robinson 2015), and of the fluidities of sexuality (Richards et al. 2017) began to make their way into popular culture (Queerstralia 2023) alongside hashtag activism such as Rainbow History Class on Australian

QueerTok (Zhou 2022). Emboldened, voices missing from mainstream culture began to assert themselves in the arts sector through unique expressions of identity politics even as neo-liberalism was seeping into pockets of the culture at large.

Government-funded partnership practices of community art and cultural development from the 1980s have been recently more theorised as socially engaged or community-centred art. This shift attended to an effort of artists to move away from colonial development framings to more self-determined examination of local concerns and culturally specific expressions and celebrations of *difference*. These practices typically aim to bring unshared narratives and underserved communities to the fore (Hawkins 1989; Badham 2010, 2019). However, such beneficent philanthropic gestures and government investment in the arts and social inclusion demanded measurement and evaluation of *impact* in return.

Language can be fraught. What is under the spotlight here goes by many names with Clare Bishop offering "socially engaged arts, community-based art, experimental communities, dialogic art, littoral art, participatory, interventionist, research-based, or collaborative art" (2006, 1) as viable nomenclature. The Dictionary app conflates *evaluation* with the "making of a judgement about the amount, number or value of something".[1] Just as vexing is *impact,* which, as Badham and others have argued (Badham 2010; Bishop 2012; Walmsley 2013), can be a coverall and euphemism for instrumental outcomes towards economic, social, or cultural "public good" (see also Bennett 2010; Gray 2009). Research has further identified the problem of evaluation by agencies with vested interests, as well as logistical difficulties in conducting audience-based and user-focused evaluations in real world contexts. This is further complicated, as Johanson and Glow have observed, by a "positive evaluation" phenomenon, in which responses affirm audience/participants' "belief in the values they perceive to be encapsulated in the cultural experience itself" (2015, 255).

The impact rubric also presumes immediate effects of art that may in fact require extended periods of time to do their work. Badham argues that the language of impact is not productive (2019, 207) not just because of its imputed violence, but also because the impact of art on individuals and communities is inevitably subtle, unpredictable, and

[1] Apple Inc. 2005–2023. Dictionary (2.3.0) App Store. https://www.dictionary.com accessed 3 July 2025.

sometimes slow working. Causality here is all but impossible to prove or document, with John Holden arguing that reductive evaluations mask what is valuable (2004, 14), while Arlene Goldbard views them as a mismatch of methods when she writes, "This quantifiable approach to value does not serve us, does nothing to advance our campaign for pluralism, participation and equity in community life" (2015, 4).

For decades, evaluation has been entangled or at the very least conflated within this web of language and aspirational objectives via mandated and transactional reporting processes that do little more than quantify funding policy outcomes. Acquittals to funders or annual reports serve as positive outcome narratives to stakeholders but many lack a nuanced relevance or application for improving the practices they report upon. There may be the occasional scraping of data sets and statistical information by external assessment agencies, but most such mechanisms are designed around ideas of accountability and within this, validation of an exchange of pre-ordained outcomes for civic largesse. Such outward-facing, post-event, bookkeeping processes create few opportunities to fold learnings back into the creative practices and community partnerships they intend to measure. More than this, critical review frameworks and impact measurement in the arts industry typically lump together multiple discreet phases (development, engagement, impact), whereas socially engaged making approaches "privilege a particular element (democracy, context, dialogue) and subsequently endorse a hierarchy of values which *should result in a corresponding unique evaluative framework*" (Badham 2019, 207, emphasis added).

The Coming Back Out Ball and LGBTIQ+ Elders Dance Club are collaborative modes of *ensemblesque* performance which foreground cooperation between diverse parties. Because of the inherent relational and responsive creative process of All The Queens Men, these collaborative projects have qualities of spontaneity and liveness that make them unpredictable. They are often modular, making parts of them unrehearsable. The "art" of these performances lies within their curation, with its etymological links of this term to cultures of care.

We however argue, punfully, that the queer community is *party-coloured*, so for these reasons, to reflect upon or assess All The Queens Men's creative outcomes requires polyphonically queered, playful, celebratory, and socially integrated approaches that open safe evaluation environments in which listening, dialogue, trust, time, and people centredness are key. Desired outcomes of All The Queens Men experiences include

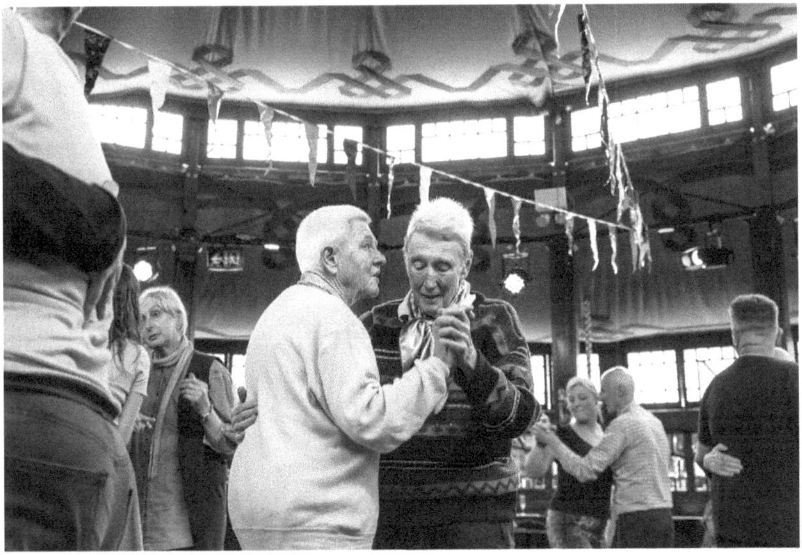

Fig. 4.2 LGBTIQ+ Elders dance club by All The Queens Men, Melbourne. Image by Bryony Jackson (2019)

subtle things, slowly emergent over time, such as enhanced sociability, enhanced intergenerational connectedness, lateral transmission of stories and knowhow, more confidence in public expressions of various aesthetics, and assertions of queer subcultures. But how do we measure these? (Fig. 4.2)

Part Three: In Which We Propose *Queevaluation* as a Speculative Values Framework Reflecting the Multivalent Nature of All The Queens Men's Processes and Outcomes

As others have observed, when socially engaged or participatory arts practices are primarily assessed on agreed objectives such as ethical criteria, or on cultural beneficence such as social inclusion, questions of authorship may be renounced and matters of aesthetics may be sidelined (Johanson and Glow 2018), while artists may be viewed as being lesser, albeit more generous, than their peers in the mainstream. We argue instead for a community-based, self-determined yet multivalent, creative approach to locating the value and values of communities and stakeholders in socially engaged arts practice. Our research partnership between artists, community, and researchers, we propose, models inherent "value" in its intergenerational, intersectional, and intercultural creative practices. More than this, we aim to align methodologies of care, self-determination, and dialogue within the offer of *queevaluation* as a counterpoint to the potential damage that may be meted out by scientism and metrics. *Queevaluation* is more than a portmanteau of "queer" and "evaluation" but an enactment of a methodology of queering (Campbell et al. 2023) that informs and underscores our inquiry. It is a posture of slow time, ethics, care, and empathy with capacity to illuminate unexpected sites and sources of "value" and "values" such projects may be harbouring or already returning to its community.

On these grounds, it will not surprise readers that the initial participatory evaluation of The Coming Back Out Ball in 2017 asked unexpected questions including: "In what ways can evaluation become a productive exchange of value and values between collaborators? And how might these processes become integrated in practice and strengthen both social and artistic outcomes?" (Badham et al. 2017). Here we see attention paid to other benchmarks such as enhanced participation and the consolidation of community, as well as professional satisfactions for artists lodged within iterative cycles of participant engagement. This allowed them to commit to their practice within a de facto site of professional development and find personal and creative fulfilment through liberation from judgement and a process-versus-outcome focus.

The measures adopted also aimed to subvert the violence of *impact* and *output* rhetoric and seek out processes that were anti-oppressive and emancipatory. It hardly bears reiterating that the queer community has specific needs and priorities: safety and freedom of assembly being foundational. Members of alphabet communities and queer-identifying artists have been subjects of study, speculation, and derision, not to mention generational trauma due to histories of violence or exclusion, imprisonment, conversion therapies, scientific experimentation, and pathologising research. To address this, collectivising rituals that foster communitas, joyful encounters, and cycles of reciprocal exchange are offered at every juncture (Murray et al. 2022). All The Queens Men's events are designed to be "accommodating of meaningful irreverence, secular ritual and affording a kind of intentional expansiveness that promotes and cultivates queer kinship" (Murray et al., 4).

Marnie Badham arrived at the adjective ***multivalent*** to capture what is needed to conduct meaningful and appropriate processes within and across this sector. Multivalent is defined in the Dictionary.com app as "having or susceptible of many applications, interpretations, meanings or values" (no date). This concept affords clearance of metricising or *intrinsically political* cultural measurement tools, with likely blind spots and biases. Multivalence moves towards a culture in which the edges between observers and participants are blurred and real relationships fostered. Within such contexts, deep listening and genuine immersion emerge to function as *activating* principles. Normative biases and expectations are sidelined in favour of embedded, cyclical, organic, and transparent modes in which both comfort and discomfort have their place, curiosity is a given, and co-creativity democratises how things are done, including how conflicts, problems, or shortfalls are identified and addressed.

Along with definitional debates, the history of socially engaged arts has been dominated by discourses of community cultural development, which seek to "contribute to civic dialogue by provoking a deeper understanding of social issues" and "by promoting community, leadership, civic dialogue, and social change" (Kelaher et al. 2014, 133) to progress "the needs of communities that are otherwise considered to be disadvantaged" (Johanson and Glow 2018, 3).

Where conventional hierarchies, temporalities, and power structures variously intrumentalise, patronise, counsel, or foreclose, All The Queens Men's *queevaluation* moves hold spaces open. All The Queens Men gatherings are meticulously crafted events that also serve as secular rites of re-connection, love, and thanksgiving. They declare and confirm queer elders' worth as pioneers, as survivors, and as individuals. Through each reiteration of such public acts they restore hope, amplify pride, and affirm LGBTIQ+ communities-within-communities with their unique culturally significant identities and needs while at the same time "shifting the way we value and create space for the older members within these communities" (Murray et al. 2022, 1).

Anecdotal reports suggest about 75% of patrons of events such as LGBTIQ+ Elders Dance Club become serial returnees. Qualitative findings garnered through one-to-one post-event interviews revealed benefits of participation that extend beyond connection and re-connection, affirmation, and pride, to include the psychosocial *impact* of eye contact and touch and health *impact* of movement along with the mood-elevating substances like dopamine and serotonin delivered by dance itself, in "triggering the reward system to release a cocktail of feelgood molecules" (Xygalatas 2022, 231). Further benefits lie in individualised expressions of identity through fashion and queer aesthetics, and in the validation bestowed by the presence of celebrities and leading lights of the arts and cultural sectors as they mix it up with the people. These have included the likes of Deborah Cheetham, Electric Fields, Yo-Yo Ma, Robyn Archer, Lois Weaver, Paul Capsis, and legendary transgender showgirl, Carlotta.

Additional feedback from individual attendees post The Coming Back Out Ball was garnered through storytelling, conversations, online surveys, and community *town hall* debriefings. The thick description (Ryle 1949; Geertz 1973) captured uplifting emotions including feelings of respect and belonging and surges of love and joy drawn forth through the "intricacies of nostalgia, memory and celebration" (Murray et al. 2022, 8).

Critically however, behind and through these emotions, other yearnings, and learnings make themselves known, combining to point towards a need for more intersectional and intergenerational engagement, more advocacy, and increased attention to the needs of LGBTIQ+ elders for better health, housing, and aged care policy across the board (Badham et al. 2017).

Part Four: In Which We Argue for Further Self-Determined Approaches to Understand the Significance and Meaning of Performance as a Tool for Care

How do you measure restored pride? What are the metrics for joy?

For many within queer communities, social connection is a key indicator of wellness and we do not need a pandemic to underscore the implications of isolation, particularly for the elderly. Scholars like Halberstam (2011) have explored how queer individuals seek out and even create alternative forms of kinship and networks of care. "Chosen" families are one example of the self-determined approaches adopted within LGBTIQ+ circles to provide psychosocial and practical support where biological families, or the state, fall short.

It is here this chapter comes in to land, proposing self-determined, co-designed evaluation practices as sites of meaning-making and of restoring democracy to culture. This counters tendencies in the arts sector to be risk averse, to yield to trends, or see data collected but not analysed or "fed back to collaborators, publicly disseminated or applied in future planning" (Badham 2019, 209). *Queevaluation* must, above all, to re-purpose Badham's words, "assess the nature and quality of something in a meaningful way" (209).

For All The Queens Men, these measures locate meaning through being expansive, generous, hope-filled, and forward-looking. For example, All The Queens Men has pioneered decentred and delegated delivery models which create opportunities for emerging local artists and cultural producers within context-specific projects. Mentorship, commitment to diversity, and the agility to pivot and hybridise when necessary have expanded the range of social enterprise models available while doing essential legacy and succession planning work to ensure sustainability for as long as the organisation has relevance, creative capacity, and demand. Furthermore, through the nuances of such relational work, including with Murray and Badham as unofficial researchers-in-residence, All The Queens Men is reframing itself, advancing a growing body of queer scholarship while making a wider contribution to socially engaged arts practice. This is not the outsourced, *fly in, fly out* model of evaluation adopted in other arenas. Research for us, like socially engaged art practice, becomes a durational art and the extended temporality of the embedded researcher makes these evaluators more likely to understand "the nuances and shifts in the social terrain" (Badham 2019, 208) and find the means to articulate them.

As part of this communitas-as-gift ethos, mentorship has become a by-product, and research is multi-purpose in sharing methodologies that upskill artists and their organisations. This has been achieved by demystifying and embedding research and reflexivity into the everyday business of the organisation so that evaluation has become a natural narrative rather than something externally imposed, to be feared.

Individuals on the All The Queens Men board of directors (past and present) have made unique contributions to establishing this narrative, bringing inclusive, and visionary approaches to the table. Jade Lillie is All The Queens Men's current chair and is renowned for cultural leadership and advocacy in championing diversity and access in the arts. Lillie's co-edited book, now in its second edition, *The Relationship is the Project* encapsulates this ethos of "process makes perfect" (2020, 11) and posits genuine collaboration as both transformational and as an art. A key area of focus for All The Queens Men's governance is to protect the Artistic

Directors from social and political harm and advocate for the power of artist-led organisations in an Australian context where artists (particularly those with community and socially engaged practices) are undervalued as leaders—a sentiment All The Queens Men Board openly rejects.

The *queevaluation* mechanisms deployed by All The Queens Men eschew one-size-fits-all toolkits that overlook the cultural complexity inherent in community relations and are attentive to "the shifts in power that co-creative projects may bring about" (Badham 2019, 207). Failure must be a possible outcome too, for, "even imperfect collaborations can offer audiences and artists great satisfaction and new experiences" (Jackson 2020, 34).

Part Five: In Which We Suggest that *Queevaluation* Fluidly Combines Empathic, Creative, Relational, and Embedded Ways of Discerning "Value" Within Safe and Reflexive Evaluation Environments

Participatory and socially engaged arts may serve as valuable PR, marketing, and community education—in All The Queens Men's case, by familiarising audiences with queer art forms and making them more approachable to communities who would otherwise keep their distance. Further values may be identified in the dialogical relationship between cross-arts practices as invigorating for the sector, and in another book chapter, it would be possible to provide evidence of how some trends in the participatory/immersive arts world have "infected" (or inflected) more conventional arts practices. There is a dialogical dynamism in play here which pushes at boundaries and asks for relevance—above and beyond diversion and entertainment—from mainstream arts. In these lights, participatory arts may be viewed as sites of research and development through prototyping gestures from which, more often, audience members are excluded.

By engaging with audiences and publics through the most formative phases of a work, preconceived notions can be overturned and expectations and ambitions expanded beyond known or familiar constraints of a given art form. At the same time transference, and even de-mystification of certain kinds of tacit knowledge, can be shared more widely. Nikos Papastergiadis offers a view of participatory practice as a cosmopolitan imaginary, "Activist, dialogical, interventionist and tactical" (2012, 155), mobilising communities around pressing social issues beyond "simple" disadvantage. Here communities become resources in their own rights, holding repositories of new thinking and lived experience. In the case of All The Queens Men, approaches to social engagement bring intergenerational cross-social colloquia opportunities that would be difficult to realise in other sites of queer culture—bars and nightclubs, dives, and festivals.

Ongoing queevaluation measures confirm that The Coming Back Out Ball and its satellite events succeed in re-engaging many queer seniors who have been experiencing isolation and open doors to ongoing relationship building and support for older people through strong social and sectoral partnerships. But as Johanson and Glow (2018, 9) have argued, the value of participatory arts practice must also go beyond community, health, and social benefits, to enrich the arts sector itself. Finally, there must be a value proposition for agility and for play—even more needed since the many pivots of the pandemic—in offering access to levity and joy that mainstream art may not so easily afford (Fig. 4.3).

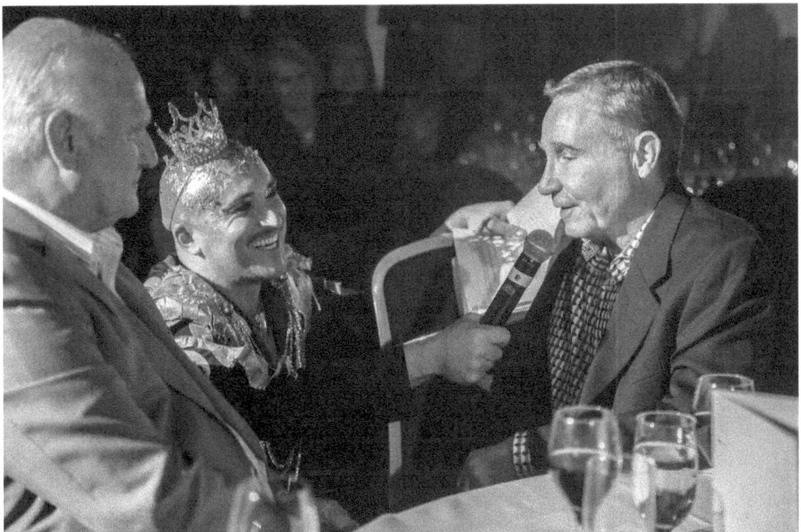

Fig. 4.3 The Coming Back Out Ball by All The Queens Men, Melbourne Town Hall. Image by Bryony Jackson (2018)

Conclusion

In response to dire news of ever-more diminished success rates for arts grant applicants (Croggon 2024; n.d.), All The Queens Men invited upon itself a new kind of evaluating gaze, in the form of the shout-out to community that is crowdsourcing. Its ask was enhanced by the allure of Plus1 prospects in which, once a goal was met, every dollar donated would be matched by Creative Australia.

Happily, targets were reached, and a doubling of the donation was secured, to confirm this pilot "campaign" a victory. This success may be read as an affirmation of complex value too, in as much as those asked responded with an excess of generosity and goodwill. This is an act of validation-by-contribution in which All The Queens Men was able to tap a sense of indebtedness and mutuality within which its community holds it. The organisation and its friends and allies have a rich and hard-won interdependency.

All The Queens Men prides itself in being a polyamorous consortium of artists and communities with a vision to unite "people of all shapes, sizes, and identities together in distinct, creative and communal experiences" (All The Queens Men website).[2] This chapter has considered how meaning and significance is created and expressed, held, and "measured" by and between artists, elders, and allies in this socially engaged arts project (Murray et al. 2022) through *queevaluation* approaches that disrupt heteronormative assumptions, and centre queer lives and queer ways of knowing. With playful openness to process and emergence, and in offering alternative principles and taxonomies of assessment that embrace non-linearity, polyphony, ambiguity, and complexity, *queevaluation* may, we contend, have wider application across the arts sector.

Queevaluation is one way of subverting calcified evaluation processes and opening integrated, safe, and equitable environments for reflection, curiosity, dialogue, and knowledge transfer. It offers alternatives in the form of a speculative value and values framework that foregrounds shared understandings of the meaning and significance of the work within what we have offered as a kind of *researcher-in-residence* partnership model. This framework, and indeed, this model, has allowed for an embedded, nuanced, and defiantly queered approach to evaluation akin to, aligned with, and reflective of the multivalent nature of All The

[2] All The Queen's Men website, https://allthequeensmen.net accessed 1May 2024.

Queens Men's creative and social processes and outcomes. It does so through the prototyping and adoption of new relational practices to the question of evaluation that prioritise and collectivise efforts to "find and make community in this time of fractured, individualized, and atomizing culture" (Harris and Holman Jones 2018, 7).

References

ABC Broadcasting. (n.d.). Episode 1: *The law. Queerstralia.* https://iview.abc.net.au/show/queerstralia Accessed 8 July 2024.

Ahmed, Sarah. 2010. Affective economies: Political feelings in Australia. *Radical Philosophy* 160: 31–38.

Albion, Astrid and Russell, Emma, K. 2022. Governing queer histories and futures: A critical place-based analysis of state apology. *Critical Criminology* 30(4), 1019–1034.

Arrow, Michelle and Angela Woollacott. 2020. Introduction—How the Personal Became Political: The Gender and Sexuality Revolutions in 1970s Australia. In *How the Personal Became Political*, 1–8. Routledge.

Badham, Marnie, Bourke, Lenine, and Meecham, Tristan. 2017. *Reflections of the Coming Back Out Ball: A dialogic evaluation.* All the Queens Men and RMIT University, https://allthequeensmen.net/wp-content/uploads/2023/04/cbob_evaluation.pdf accessed 7 July 2024.

Badham, Marnie. 2019. Spectres of evaluation indeterminacy and the negotiation of value(s) in socially engaged art. In *Co Creation* eds. Céline Poulin and Marie Preston, 5, 205–216. CAC Brétigny.

Badham, Marnie, 2010. Legitimation: The case for 'socially engaged arts'-navigating art history, cultural development and arts funding narratives. *Local-Global: Identity, Security, Community* (7) 84–99.

Barrett, Catherine, Carolyn Whyte, Jude Comfort, Anthony Lyons, and Pauline Crameri. 2025. Social connection, relationships and older lesbian and gay people. *Sexual and Relationship Therapy* 30, (1): 131–142.

Bennett, Tony. 2010. *Making culture, changing society.* Routledge.

Bishop, Clare. 2006. The social turn: Collaboration and its discontents. *Artforum*, February, 179–185.

Bishop, Clare. 2012. Artificial hells: Participatory arts and the politics of spectatorship. Verso.

Boucher, Leigh and Robert Reynolds. 2018. Decriminalisation, apology and expungement: Sexual citizenship and the problem of public sex in Victoria. *Australian Historical Studies* 49, no. 4: 457–474.

Bradway, Teagan and Freeman, ELizabeth, 2022. *Queer kinship: Race, sex, belonging, form.* Duke University Press.

Campbell, Marion May, Lawrence Macambra Ypil, Francesca Rendle-Short, Deborah Wardle, Ames Hawkins, Quinn Eades, Stayci Taylor, Peta Murray, Natalie Harkin, Natalie, Antonia Pont and Anonymous. 2023. Queering 2023 *A to Z of Creative Writing Methods*. eds. Wardle, Deborah et al. London: Bloomsbury Academic. 141-143.

Connell, Raewyn. 2009. *Gender*, Vol. 14. Polity.

Croggon, Alison. 2024. Stage plight: The state of Australian theatre. The Monthly, June, 58–62, Swartz Media.

Fela, Geraldine. 2018. Blood politics: Australian nurses, HIV and the battle for rights on the wards. *Labour History: A Journal of Labour and Social History* 115: 87–104.

Feinberg, Leslie. 2013. Transgender liberation: A movement whose time has come. *The transgender studies reader* (2013): 205–220.

Geertz, Clifford. 2008. Thick description: Toward an interpretive theory of culture. In *The cultural geography reader*, 41–51. Routledge.

Goldbard, Arlene. 2015. New creative community: The art of cultural development. New Village Press.

Gray, C. 2009. Commodification and instrumentality in cultural policy. International Journal of Cultural Policy, 13(2), 203–215.

Gray, Clive. 2007. Commodification and instrumentality in cultural policy. *International journal of cultural policy*, *13*(2), 203–215.

Halberstam, Jack. 2021 "The Queer Art of Failure." *Multitudes* 82, no. 1: 205–213.

Hawkins, Gay. 1989. Reading community arts policy: from Nimbin to the Gay Mardi Gras. *Media Information Australia*, *53*(1): 31–35.

Holden, John. 2004. Capturing cultural value: How culture has become a tool of government policy. Demos.

Holman Jones, Stacy and Daniel Harris. 2018. *Queering autoethnography*. Routledge.

Jackson, Eleonor, 2020. The art of collaboration. In *The Relationship is the Project*, eds. Lillie, Jade, Jax Jacki Brown, Kate Larsen, and Cara Kirkwood Brow Books. 33–38

Johanson, Katya and Glow, Hilary. 2015. A virtuous circle: The positive evaluation phenomenon in arts audience research. In *Participations: Journal of Audience and Reception Studies*, 12(1), 254.

Joosten, Melanie. 2017. The Coming Back Out Ball: Being out and proud and older in Australia. *The Guardian*. 25 March.

Karp, Paul. 2022. Scott Morrison defends delaying protections for LGBTQ students as party tensions resurface. *The Guardian*. 8 May.

Kelaher, Margaret, Naomi Berman, David Dunt, Victoria Johnson, Steve Curry, and Lindy Joubert. 2014. Evaluating community outcomes of participation in community arts: A case for civic dialogue. *Journal of Sociology* 50, no. 2: 132–149.

Massaquoi, Notisha. 2015. Queer theory and intersectionality. In I*nternational encyclopedia of the social and behavioural sciences* (2nd ed). Elsevier.

Mauss, Marcel. 2002. *The gift: The form and reason for exchange in archaic societies*. Routledge.

Moreton-Robinson, Aileen. 2015. *The white possessive: Property, power, and indigenous sovereignty*. University of Minnesota Press.

Murray, Peta, Adelaide Rief, Marnie Badham, Tristan Meecham, Bec Reid, and Lenine Bourke. 2022. Birds of a feather: On queerness, performance, the coming back out ball and the LGBTIQ+ elders dance club. *Australasian Drama Studies*, 81, 237–271.

Murray, Peta. 2014. Elder-flowering: Creative resistance and the theatre of endurance-or vice versa: An introduction to a research project-in-progress. *Creative Manoeuvres: Writing, Making, Being*, 157–168.

Murray, Peta. 2017. *Essayesque dismemoir: w/rites of elder-flowering* [Doctoral dissertation]. RMIT University.

Murray, Peta and Bridgid Magner. 2022. Putting the imp into imposter syndrome. In *The Palgrave handbook of imposter syndrome in higher education*. Eds. Addison, Michelle, Maddie Breeze, and Yvette Taylor: 545–562, Springer.

Papastergiadis, Nikos. 2012. *Cosmopolitanism and Culture*. John Wiley & Sons.

Rendle-Short, Francesca. 2021. Finding communitas: Encounter, unfolding, and creative writing. *TEXT: Journal of Writing and Writing Courses*, 25(2), 1–19.

Reynolds, Robert and Shirleene Robinson. 2016. Australian lesbian and gay life stories: A national oral history project. *Australian Feminist Studies*, 31(89), 363–376.

Richards, Cristina, Walter Pierre Bouman, Walter Pierre, and Meg-John Barker. 2017. *Non-binary genders*. London: Palgrave Macmillan.

Ryle, Gilbert. 1949. Concept of the mind. Hutchinson and Company.

Sendziuk, Paul. 2003. *Learning to trust: Australian responses to AIDS*. UNSW Press.

Simic, Zora. 2017. Gay and lesbian history now. *History Australia*, 14 (2), 315–321.

Theatre Network Australia. Research reports. https://tna.org.au/our-work/research-resources/research-reports/, accessed 22 June 2024.

Turner, Edith. 2012. *Communitas: The anthropology of collective joy*. Springer.

Walmsley, Ben. 2013. Co-creating theatre: Authentic engagement or inter-legitimation. *Cultural Trends*, 22(2), 108–118.

Willett, Graham. 2013. Australia: nine jurisdictions, one long struggle. *Downloaded from the Humanities Digital Library* (2013): 207.

Xygalatas, Dimitris. 2022. *Ritual: How seemingly senseless acts make life worth living*. Little, Brown Spark.
Zhou, Min. 2022. There's a new generation of queer storytelling & it's found a home on TikTok. *Refinery29*. www.refinery29.com/en-us/2022/03/10901818/queer-storytelling-tiktok, accessed 7 July 2024.

CHAPTER 5

Home Ground: Evaluating in the Liminal Space

Jacqui Moyes and Fran Kewene

The Context

> You cannot work in a community without understanding the impact of prison on women and whānau.
> (Ceila Lashlie, personal communication, Nov, 2002)

Established in 2019 as a response to the inequities, racism, trauma, addiction and mental ill health women experienced within the justice system in Aotearoa New Zealand, Home Ground delivers arts-informed projects addressing the issues women and whānau face. Aotearoa New Zealand is a small island nation located in the Pacific with a current population of just over 5 million people. Colonised by Great Britain in the 1800s through acts of violence, warfare, land confiscations, cultural subjugation

J. Moyes (✉) · F. Kewene
Wellington, New Zealand
e-mail: Jacqui@homegroundnz.com

F. Kewene
e-mail: fran.kewene@vuw.ac.nz

M. Mullen et al. (eds.), *Artful Evaluation for Creative Health and Wellbeing*, New Directions in Cultural Policy Research,
https://doi.org/10.1007/978-3-032-17063-7_5

and oppression, Māori (the Indigenous peoples) are now a minority on their own lands. Māori experience inequities, marginalisation and racism entrenched in contemporary acts of Eurocentric legislative legitimisation (George and Ngamu 2020). Aotearoa New Zealand is a society where the economic gap between the haves and have-nots has grown, and where women, children and the elderly experience disparities built on the political ideologies of neoliberalism (Workman and McIntosh 2013).

In Aotearoa New Zealand, most women inside prison have family outside, with more than 23,000 children across Aotearoa New Zealand having a parent in prison. Māori make up only 17.3% of the population with Māori women only slightly outnumbering Māori men. Māori are a young population, with the median ages for males and females being 25.8 and 27.9, respectively, compared with non-Māori, whose median ages are 37.0 and 39.0 years, respectively.[1] Māori women, however, are more likely to be sent to prison than non-Māori women, comprising 63% of the female prison population (Fryers 2018). It is, therefore, essential to position the development and implementation of Home Ground's projects in collaboration with Māori, centring Māori concepts and values into practice to meet the needs of Māori women. Home Ground also understands their responsibilities and obligations to te Tiriti o Waitangi. Te Tiriti o Waitangi, one of Aotearoa New Zealand's founding documents, is a treaty of settlement between the British Crown and the sovereign nations Tino Rangatiratanga o ngā iwi o Nu Tireni (the absolute leaders of the tribes of New Zealand) (Mutu 2011). This Māori language treaty outlines the rightness of obligations between the British representatives of the Crown and the sovereignty of Māori leaders over their lands and peoples. The intent of te Tiriti o Waitangi was never realised. Māori continue to seek redress through the Waitangi Tribunal, a permanent commission of inquiry established under the Treaty of Waitangi Act 1975, which adjudicates claims brought by Māori relating to historical breaches of te Tiriti o Waitangi. The reality of this colonial legacy is the over-representation of Māori in prisons, with incarceration engendering an oppressive experience that is inherently violent, which leads to a total disruption of family, housing, income and health. In *The power of mothers: Releasing our children* Celia Lashlie (2010), a former prison officer, social justice advocate

[1] Statistics New Zealand. 2023. *Māori population estimates: At 30 June 2023*. https://www.stats.govt.nz/information-releases/maori-population-estimates-at-30-june-2023/.

and author, highlights the often overlooked experience of the incarcerated woman, noting:

> We never pause to ask what she wants; we never take time to look at her life through her eyes; and we never consider the possibility that success in her life will not, and does not need to, look like success in ours. (174)

This chapter considers what success might look like from the perspective of incarcerated women engaged in participatory arts. It seeks to explore the liminal space of evaluation; evaluation between the funders' and artists' practice, and the tension that exists between art and creativity and art for health and wellbeing. The chapter aims to pause and take time in the liminal space to explore the tensions which exist for women in the justice system with regard to consent and coercion; in prison life, home life, living back in community and in women's relationships with whānau, and with themselves. We document the whakapapa (genealogy) of Home Ground, its evaluation style and the liminal spaces of evaluation with their community of artists, with their arts-informed practice, with their funders and with the women in the justice system. Artistic Director Jacqui Moyes and Indigenous Health Academic/Applied Theatre Deviser Fran Kewene combine their collective experience in this chapter to examine and explore the intersection and liminality of arts, justice and evaluation within the context of Aotearoa New Zealand.

Home Ground

Take Your (*liminal*)Time
We work in a space of holding on
Struggling to come up from the white wash of our minds
Where joy is felt in moments of freedom
Obliviating the past takes some strong chemicals and self-harm
Sometimes even Prison

The pre-interview is a phone call,
a conversation at the kitchen table:

> "It's my first hand out of drowning and I'm ready"
> "I'm not a criminal, I'm a drunk driver"

How do we measure what we do? If we aren't 'them'
How do we stay well when we do what we do? If we are 'them'
We can measure what we want, write down numbers in any way
Like the current government measuring how many people they get off a benefit
Death and prison are a bonus in this space.

The evaluation is in so many noisy strands
Woven together with the wishes of
actions
not words.

The constant measurement of the artists, facilitators, and women
But never the context we work in
This is the challenge for change
in the stories that we speak.

Actions speak louder
than words.

This poem written by Jacqui Moyes, founder and Creative Director of Home Ground, is a provocation, a challenge, the opening to what Home Ground is and how they evaluate in challenging liminal spaces. Liminal spaces are considered in this chapter to be like the transition between prison and community which offer opportunities for growth and change. Where identity and belonging can be redefined. In these liminal spaces critical choices are made, and boundaries blur between power, control and personal agency. This is why consent is so important to our work and the evaluative process. The key to practice and evaluation in these transitional liminal spaces is making the gaps and grey areas visible, while maintaining hope and embracing the potential for healing and empowerment.

I (Jacqui) was lucky enough to grow up with dance and discover the power of community performing arts as an 'at-risk' teenager. After many years of getting in trouble, travelling throughout Aotearoa New Zealand, Australia, the United States, Canada and the United Kingdom and performing as a busker, I returned to Aotearoa New Zealand to get a Bachelor of Arts in Education and Gender Studies at Te Herenga Waka Victoria University Wellington. After meeting social justice advocate and author Celia Lashlie in a Criminology lecture, I followed Celia's guidance and ended up working across a range of roles within the justice sector as an arts educator in prisons and Youth Justice Residencies, providing arts mentoring support to whānau in social services and as the national Arts in Corrections Advisor. With a strong belief in using creative experiences as a tool to build connected communities, my current focus is on strengthening support for women and their whānau in the justice system through the Home Ground projects.

I first encountered Fran Kewene via her kaupapa-Māori headphone theatre when actor Julie Edwards was invited to perform scenes from Fran's one-woman play *Barrier Ninja* (Kewene 2017) in the very first Home Ground project. *Barrier Ninja* is an Indigenous headphone theatre play which has woven together nine very personal stories, from medical professionals through to people dealing with health issues, while navigating the health system. It has been seen by over 1,000 medical students, used as a tool to explore arts-based research methodology, health equity and service delivery within Fran's university teaching, and performed in a number of theatre fringe festivals throughout Aotearoa New Zealand. On seeing *Barrier Ninja,* I was excited by the honest, kind and authentic description of the challenges faced by whānau in the health system. Women who witnessed this performance had a shared understanding of this very real experience of racism and systemic inequities. When someone sees their experience represented as part of a shared performance event, they might accept that systemic challenges such as racism, sexism and state violence are something that many people face, not just them alone.

Home Ground started when Jacqui was working in prisons, creating devised theatre and, at the same time, unpacking her own personal trauma, dislocation and feelings of not belonging. Many women have been told they are stupid, worthless, will never amount to anything and are far from creative. Creative opportunities challenge these beliefs, giving women the platform to change the world, starting from their own kitchen table. Home Ground, therefore, creates space for women in the justice system to pause, nurture hope, activate social change and create better lives for themselves and future generations. They achieve this through co-designed and created projects with the women who have experienced the justice system. The women have the opportunity to identify art forms that are relevant to them and their whānau and be responsive to the constant social change. This means Home Ground measures and evaluates their projects in a way that keeps their values and guiding principles, their tikanga (correct procedure), in focus while they carve out a space for themselves and the community they work with in a colonial, capitalist, Eurocentric society.

Home Ground uses creative multi-disciplinary arts practice, such as theatre, dance, creative writing and Indigenous art-practices, such as taonga pūoro (Māori cultural wind instruments) and waiata (songs), so that women can tap into their own way of expressing themselves and so that they can pass these forms of self-expression on to their whānau when at home. We all deserve to feel valued, to have a voice, to be heard and understood. With a deeper understanding of our stories, and therefore ourselves, we are more able to weave into our community. As our society and community learn and understand our stories, we are more able to work together to create social change. Through collaborations, we can create opportunities to amplify the voices of people affected by the justice system and start these tough conversations (Fig. 5.1).

Home Ground's projects, which take place both inside and outside prison, consistently ask the system, and the women who live inside that system, to pause and ask for what they want, to listen to their voices, to

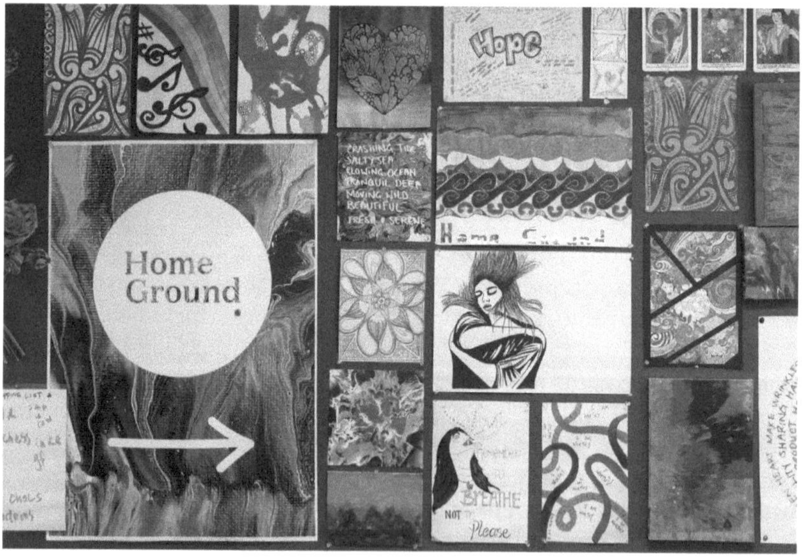

Fig. 5.1 Hearts on display. Artwork created by women who have participated in a variety of Home Ground projects. Photo credit: Rebecca McMillan (2024)

reflect upon what lived experience can offer and what skills they have to adjust to the world outside and become active citizens. Home Ground, through its art-informed practice, enables these women to speak for themselves, to tell their truth, to create the art that can tell their own story. Home Ground is there to support women to find a sense of belonging after prison, and maybe even in prison, but it provides a constant reminder that prison is not a home.

Home Ground's prison-based programmes, developed over five years, aim to provide respite in the system, space to be human, a holiday from prison reality and a moment to let women's souls shine. It creates a liminal space in which the competing pressures on the women can be held at bay for a moment in time. Meanwhile, the community-based projects provide a bridge after prison back to the community where women hopefully learn how to carve out space for themselves to practise healthy boundaries and rediscover who they are beyond institutionalisation. On all Home Ground projects, women work towards surrounding themselves and their whānau with a strong creative community no matter where their home is, whether in prison or back in the community. They take the time and space to ask themselves;

Who are you?
What do you want?
To say No.

Do No Harm

Grounded in the context of Aotearoa New Zealand, Home Ground firstly acknowledges mana whenua (Māori, the Indigenous people of Aotearoa), the people of this land and place. Home Ground, within their practice, responds to the cultural diversity of its artists and women by drawing on the knowledge and expertise held within the group through sourcing waiata and karakia (blessings). Māori and Pacific representation from artists and facilitators also matters to Home Ground. We are mindful that facilitators are from a range of cultural backgrounds and aim to be inclusive, but are aware, as a te Tiriti o Waitangi partner, we have limitations in the knowledge and practice of te ao Māori (Māori perspective). Home Ground prioritises establishing long-term and equitable relationships with artist practitioners, with the intent of sharing and exchanging knowledge and skills.

Faced with the many systemic barriers which surround our work Home Ground responds to these challenges through embedding and enacting our values, which ground and focus the development, implementation and evaluation of our projects. These values are:

- Creativity matters
- Do no harm
- Nothing about us without us
- Honour the wisdom of lived experience
- Strength through connectedness
- Trust the process

Home Ground also takes a people-centred approach to our mahi (work), so that women and whānau can benefit from accessible programming. For example, workshops are scheduled during school hours and term time. Contracted artists are not expected to work during school holidays, and can prioritise whānau first. Their practice aims to be reflective, respectful, and humble, especially when engaging with all people with diverse cultural identities. Jacqui utilises Māori tikanga principles that have been gifted to her and learnt in relationship with individual Māori and Māori communities such as myself (Fran). These tikanga principles informed by Māori knowledge are the spine on which the daily rituals and activities within the projects unfold. Rituals such as opening and closing the day with karakia are woven seamlessly into the structure of the programme, embedding manaakitanga (hospitality) and whanaungatanga (relationships) into practice, which acknowledges the different ways in which we can relate to one another. Manaakitanga means lots of things, caring for people and supporting people, but for Home Ground, it means engaging with all people to ensure that the mana (authority) of a person is upheld. Poroaki (farewell) is a way to close the intensive phase of the project with a process of sharing and leaving the day there, in that moment in time and space, followed by closing the day with karakia. Home Ground has no fixed model of practice and evaluation, but these processes are always grounded in a collectivist ideology rather than individualism, as is their approach to developing community. These practices acknowledge that Home Ground works together for the betterment of everyone. Home Ground's obligation to be in relationship with mana whenua also means they need to build their own knowledge and be culturally competent (Smith 2014; Smith and Smith 2019).

Finding the Money

Home Ground started with a $4,000 prize from the Sonja Davies Peace Award in 2019 and a $1,000 philanthropic gift from Heather and Brian Main. Home Ground put together a hefty proposal that was turned down by the prisons due to a lack of capacity to deliver it. Then, the New Zealand Probation Service contributed $10,000 for the very first pilot project in the community. Previously, Jacqui had worked as the National Arts in Corrections Advisor, which meant having strong existing relationships in the corrections and arts communities. The prison director of Arohata Women's Prison was an active champion of the arts, and the regional manager of Probation Services, who believed in the potential of Home Ground, signed off on a pilot programme Kahukura (is red ochre, but is the clay from which the first Māori women was formed and life breathed into her). The name Kahukura was chosen to reflect the potential we all have for freedom and transformation and that the red cloak of lived experience can be worn with pride.

Home Ground's journey with Creative New Zealand (CNZ), the national arts funding and development agency, also began in 2019 with the intention of strengthening Home Ground as a multi-disciplinary community arts initiative. Home Ground applied for a CNZ Arts Grant for three projects to create a sustainable body of work, to be able to train up artists and to acknowledge the workload involved in individual applications and the reporting process. Quite radically at the time, CNZ gave Home Ground enough funding to deliver the three projects in a year. Home Ground aimed to make arts participation more accessible to New Zealanders, and to train artists to work safely with women in the justice system. Their evaluation shifted from evaluations tailored for the funder to evaluation that included understanding the artists' experiences of working with Home Ground as well as artistic outcomes.

This shift is important because, at the time in 2019, Home Ground sat in a liminal space between two worlds. The world of prisons and probation, where there needed to be a health or clinical outcome, and the world of 'The Arts', where art was not understood to be intrinsically linked to health and community development. Also, Home Ground was dancing on a line of creativity rather than 'The Arts', striving to be a process-driven project with professional artistic outcomes. This meant multiple funding applications, multiple reports and extensive advocacy for creativity to be seen as something that matters to a very specific community of women and their whānau. At this time, funders were not covering administrative hours, so all of the pre- and post-grant work fell on the Creative Director. Like any working artist, multiple other contracts were, and still are, necessary to pay the bills and to independently fund the work, even when funders are funding.

Home Ground then secured funding from the Ministry of Women along with stronger support from CNZ and the Department of Corrections, who agreed to split the bill on the larger annual projects. When COVID-19 hit, Home Ground was one of the many arts organisations that moved online. They eventually secured a larger, three-year Manatū Taonga Ministry of Culture and Heritage Creative Arts Recovery and Employment Fund, which was established when arts funding was significantly uplifted for a fixed time during the pandemic.

For every different funder, there was a different type of funding application process and method of reporting, different contractual obligations, key performance indicators (KPIs), evaluation tools and reporting expectations. The accountability and pressure of funders' reporting motivates Home Ground to collect strong data, take great images and frame it all with a participant consent process right at the very beginning of any engagement. With so many different ways of working, KPIs and outcomes, the evaluation process has been extensive. Home Ground has implemented so many ways of evaluating that six years later they can fill clouds with feedback forms.

Institutional limitations often dictate the changing shape of a project, and new evaluation practice is also needed to reflect that. This constant evolution of evaluation means that Home Ground has developed specific practices that are consistent with the values mentioned earlier and are now embedded in the project framework.

Evaluation is Consensual

Evaluation is a process we do every day. We make judgements and assess the worth, merit, or value of what we did and how we did it. Evaluation is, therefore, built on the beliefs and values of the people who assess the worth of what was done and how it was done. It is a retrospective process, intent on understanding what has been done and, hopefully, what can be learnt from that doing to improve or replicate similar activities (Moewaka Barnes 2009). The art of evaluation, as seen by Home Ground, is the telling of the stories that make up the work that they do. Ideally, it is an honest reflection of their practice as experienced by everyone involved. It is also a way to figure out what could be done better, and how it might be done differently. The evaluative process includes critical analysis of how the women practise with the guidance and support of tuakana (elder brother of a male, elder sister of a female, cousin of the same gender from a more senior branch of the family) who understand the diversity of mātauranga Māori (Māori knowledge), as they deliver programmes around the country. Tuakana, in the Home Ground context, are the women who have completed projects and stay on to become project facilitators.

The very first pilot project, Kahukura was evaluated to discover what worked. To test all of the contract criteria against practice, so as to create something with women rather than for women. Home Ground asked: Was it relevant and engaging? Was it for women by women? Was it trauma-informed? These questions were tested through qualitative and quantitative measures. Creative and clinical practice were merged to create evaluation techniques that were participatory, rather than relying on questionnaires. A majority of the measuring was focused on self-reflection in the creative/project space in real time, unpacking processes through artwork and reflective group discussions.

Home Ground found that as the projects' funders changed, they started evaluating more to meet the funders' criteria and KPIs. The learning over five years has been to strike a balance, collect the data that is necessary for funders and partners and prioritise the information to keep delivery aligned with guiding principles. Consent is the key to the balancing act of evaluation for the funders and evaluation for assessing principles alignment. It is another liminal space, determining value and worth between the measures of the funder's requests and Home Ground's own values and principles.

Seeking Consent

When a woman signs up to a Home Ground programme, information is gathered that is necessary for funders, such as basic demographic information, their Probation Officer, attendance and outcomes for participating.

But Home Ground also asks questions which humanise the individual such as the name that they prefer to be called. Often the system name is different from their chosen name. How do they choose to identify? Because when Home Ground uses the description 'women', they mean anyone who identifies as a woman or as non-binary. Women are asked if they give permission to use their data—and often they do not.

Home Ground actively challenges traditional hierarchical power structures in arts practice by involving artists and communities in decision-making processes. Consent, collaboration and co-creation are central to the approach, allowing artists and participants to reclaim agency and challenge dominant narratives. The story that society, the media and politicians tell about women in the justice system, is one of individual blame and shame, not systemic failings. Home Ground believes the stories we tell matter. They are inherently political. During Home Ground projects, systemic racism is explored, sexism is confronted and we highlight the role of capitalism in the colonial project.

Home Ground participants who have transitioned into co-facilitators, tuakana and emerging artists, reflect on the importance of internal advocacy. These wāhine believe that contributing to the korero (speak) is a form of advocacy, internally and externally, where they can work towards social change. They acknowledge that being honest about the reality of the lives they have lived can be challenging, but using creative approaches can help to unravel and reshape the narratives they have of themselves, and their life experiences. This truth is neither good nor bad but is the ability to be honest about their needs, as this is what prison takes away from you. A liminal space of holding two worlds at the same time, the world of the prison and the world of community. By centring the experiences and needs of individuals in challenging contexts such as prison, we can humanise women in the justice system and influence the people in positions of power that make the decisions that affect their lives.

Enacting Consent

> *You came in as people and spoke to us as people. It's a simple thing but it's not, cos it never happens.*
> Project Rua Prison Participant, 2021, written evaluation feedback

The most powerful evaluative practice Home Ground does is asking participants what they think, listening to it and then acting on it. We believe that women choosing to participate and having the power to say no is essential to the programme because it gives them power back over their lives. The Home Ground programme was co-designed with women in the room, so the practice model has co-creation in its bones. Every day, we ask, 'What can we do better?'.

The evaluation methods of Home Ground are embedded in daily rituals. There are many opportunities for participants to be honest about their experience of the projects, probation service, their partners, prison life, kids! Authenticity is encouraged, as is radical acceptance of where participants are right now so that they can work towards who or how they want to be.

The work is created to be relevant and fun, to provide representation and to create an opportunity to amplify voices. Asking for feedback, measuring outcomes and carving out space for reflection is how Home Ground improves delivery and practice. However, there are three distinct strands which create tension for practitioners like Home Ground in their relationship with evaluation. These three strands are: evaluating practice as artists; evaluation of the work to ensure the community is experiencing the work in the way it was intended; and funder-driven evaluations. This tension is reflected in the liminal space they exist in, straddling multiple thresholds such as:

- Art/wellbeing
- Community/Prisons
- Institution/Freedom
- Consent/Coercion
- Creative/Clinical
- Resistance/Resilience

Home Ground asks women to step into a creative liminal space, to trust the collective process and unpack what they want, when they want. Home Ground provides the space, and participants can take the time that is right for them. Timing is everything, and consent is everything else.

Evaluation and the Notion of Self as Change Maker

Home Ground uses evaluation as a tool to create change, not just assess whether change has happened. Our interpretation of evaluation is that it involves tools that speak to everyone, it has visual elements, a purpose and an opportunity to tell a story that reflects who we are. As artists and practitioners, one of Home Ground's good practice principles is to understand and support the context they are working in. Home Ground believes we all have different places to occupy on the wheel of social change and believes that an understanding of where you stand will inform your practice. From the three strikes sentencing law (which aims to deter repeat offenders with a second strike that means no parole, and for a third strike offenders will have to serve the maximum penalty without parole) to prison abolition, artists need to understand the context and know why they do the work they do.

Good practice for Home Ground looks like prioritising working in partnership while finding opportunities for change making, seeking clarity around why and how we advocate. Simultaneously, Home Ground believes in prison abolition and system change, which is why Home Ground works as a collective, as it is safer and maintains accountability. Working in partnership with larger organisations is critical to finding opportunities for advocacy. Good communication between partners can provide strategic clarity around how to advocate for system change.

To activate the self-belief that a person can change the environment they spend time in, Home Ground begins each day with the group writing out objectives on the whiteboard in colourful markers. As a group, they collectively write a list of what they want to get out of the day, or a workshop. Guest artists are involved in this conversation as well. Then, at the end of the day, as part of a 30-minute reflection process, everyone is asked how they did with the objectives—asking questions such as: 'Do you think we met our objectives?', 'What did we do well?' and 'What could we do differently?' If, for example, someone says they want more music played, that can be done the next day. If they had a negative experience in the probation van, the problem can be unpacked, and the collective can try to resolve it. This navigation takes experience and guidance, especially in a prison system full of hierarchical decision-making.

The Home Ground projects take place in two distinct environments creating a liminal space of resilience and resistance for the artists who come on the projects, for Home Grounds permanent facilitators and for the women who join the projects. Creative resilience can be found peacefully, whereas creative resistance must be explored carefully in the Prison space. When women are in a position of powerlessness, it is not productive to highlight that, they know it already, and the artist is a tourist in this space. Home Ground uses creative practice to articulate the experience of incarceration so that women can see that two truths do, in fact, exist. They may have done 'bad' things, but they can simultaneously be good people, capable of creating beautiful works of art.

Reflecting on the Home Ground journey so far, Home Ground has identified that it is important to document the methodology. This means articulating the process for the facilitators and not making assumptions that osmosis will happen. Artists involved in projects need to know where the pou (pillar) are and what are the evaluation practices. They need to know the non-negotiables.

The Lei Evaluation Tool

A lei (a garland or wreath of objects strung together, often flowers, that is worn as a necklace) is a symbol of peace, love, friendship, celebration and honour. Home Ground uses the structure of a lei as a tool for evaluation and self-reflection. The lei created over time becomes a collaborative artwork. At the end of each day during a project, a different coloured paper flower is offered to everyone. They choose their own colour and pen. The choice seems simple and small, but this practice embeds and reinforces the consensual process and empowerment for the women to make personal choices. The lei is also an opportunity for self-reflection. Everyone is given the same prompt by someone in the group, an artist or participant. For example, 'write down the best thing you got out of today'. The individuals take time to choose a word or phrase that reflects how the day has gone for them and write it on the paper flower. Everyone's flowers are then threaded onto the lei, which grows into a collective piece as the work continues. Over the year, in all of the different spaces, prison and community, the lei gathers and holds the intentional energy of all of the people who contribute to the projects. The lei has become a daily ceremony of belonging, for every participant, artist and practitioner to make their mark on the story of Home Ground (Fig. 5.2).

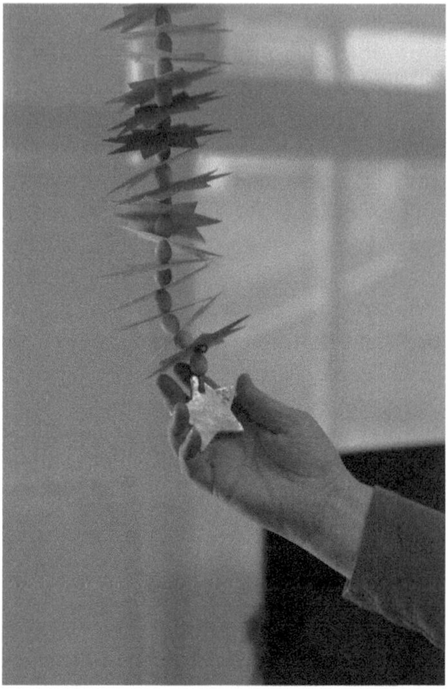

Fig. 5.2 Home Ground evaluation lei. Photo credit: Rebecca McMillan (2024)

COVID-19 Pivot: The Evolution of More Evaluation Tools

COVID-19 lockdowns and ongoing disruption to services forced Home Ground to radically adapt to a new normal. Home Ground needed to create a response to barriers that prevented the crew from being able to provide in-person projects to wāhine inside and outside prison. In the community, online delivery was essential, but then, women who had experienced the justice system were often experiencing a digital divide. For example, internet access was not good in regional areas, or they were working off their cell phones. Printed material became essential again, as no one in the prison had face-to-face options or online access, and women in the community were struggling to carve out space at home. The answer was a bespoke creative workbook. The workbook consolidates the spirit of Home Ground into a tangible, remote tool that can act as a creative sanctuary for participants. Featuring rituals, an abundant use of colour, a sense of community and artistic collaborations with the creative whānau.

The evaluative practices have shown some of the benefits of the workbook, including: celebrating the creative journey of participants by showcasing participants' artwork; maintaining connection to Home Ground between projects; being a resource to use in the weekly online sessions; revising the learnings from in-person Home Ground projects; creative prompts to extend participant's art practice; a resource for wāhine to share exercises with their whānau to create collaborations; and a tool for managing big emotions when experiencing isolation in the prison or in the community.

Professional Artists and Evaluation

After five years of growth, development and adaptation, Home Ground's evaluation methodology is integral to our practice and can be understood as intentional praxicality, the cycle of action, practice and reflection. Through the process of praxicality, theory is practice-informed, and practice is theory-informed (Smith 2014). This cycle is about constant learning and improvement through doing and reflecting with people who are affected by the work. It is personified in the notion of akoako (to consult together), a continued cycle of teaching and learning and adjusting. The professional artists are still visible in the process, not hidden. They perform, contribute to the creation of works and collaborate.

The participants who transition into the tuakana role have to navigate changing relationship dynamics. It can be a turbulent time, and guidance and clarity are needed in this transition. When we collectively grow it is often the unstructured moments that shape us. We have learnt from experience that a conversation over a smoke break can ruin relationships, that our vulnerabilities can break our confidence, when relationships and confidence are needed more than ever. So much more care is needed in this transition process, for all involved. What is seen as an opportunity is also a hurdle.

Working in the justice system with participants who have experienced serious trauma can elicit trauma responses for artists, especially those with lived experience of the justice system. Home Ground takes the responsibility of artist care seriously and aims to provide as much support as necessary to maintain wellbeing. Inductions, training and a strong debriefing practice is part of working with Home Ground. This responsibility includes financial reciprocity, and being paid fairly for work that is, at times, incredibly demanding.

Poroaki—Farewell

Home Ground aims to create a supportive and inclusive work and practice environment that recognises the value and potential of every team member, participant and artist. Our hope is to foster a sense of community and connectedness among team members and empower women in the justice system to activate social change through utu (reciprocity), giving and taking, the balance. Reciprocal exchange. Through five years of creative projects, Home Ground has contributed to empowering more than 200 women and collaborated with over 40 artists.

Ideally, Home Ground will always take the time that is needed to develop relationships and connections with the women they work with, organisational partnerships and the arts community that collaborates on projects. A slowburn approach that encourages reflection on the design of practice, with considered delivery to respond to constant social change, often goes against the usual pressure cooker style of community arts and culture projects. There is a delicate balance of intentions between practice, lived experience and funding-driven outcomes in these liminal spaces. The main challenge Home Ground encounters in our practice is navigating and delivering in an overstretched prison system that has become used to extended periods of lockdown.

Home Ground will continue to evaluate in a creative way to keep the values and guiding principles, our tikanga, in focus. Evaluation in the liminal space is essential, as it allows us to acknowledge and name the gaps and challenges in women's lives, across multiple thresholds. It prioritises listening to what they have to say about how they persevere in carving out creative space in a colonial, capitalist, Eurocentric society. It is in these magical gaps and spaces between the worlds we walk in—that hope and a sense of belonging are possible.

References

Fryers, Andy. 2018. Crime and punishment. Stuff. https://interactives.stuff.co.nz/2018/05/prisons/crime.html/. Accessed 1 July 2024

George, Lily, and Elaine, Ngamu. 2020. Te Piringa Poho: Healing, potential and transformation for Māori women. In *Neo-colonial injustice and the mass imprisonment of indigenous women*, ed. Lily George, Adele N. Norris, Antje Deckert, and Juan Tauri, 239–267. Cham, Switzerland: Palgrave Macmillan. https://doi.org/10.1007/978-3-030-44567-6_12

Kewene, Francis W. 2017. Verbatim and Maori Theatre Techniques: Documenting People's Experiences of Hauora (Doctoral dissertation, University of Otago). University of Otago. https://hdl.handle.net/10523/7028. Accessed 5 March 2025

Lashlie, Celia. 2010. *The power of mothers: Releasing our children*. Auckland: HarperCollins

Moewaka Barnes, Helen. 2009. The evaluation hikoi: A Maori overview of programme evaluation. Auckland: Te Ropu Whariki

Mutu, Margaret. 2011. *The state of Māori rights*. Wellington: Huia

Smith, Graham Hingangaroa. 2014. Transforming research: The emerging kaupapa Māori research context in Aotearoa. Australian Association for Research in Education. https://www.aare.edu.au/assets/documents/MAIN_Transforming_Research_NZARE_2014.pdf. Accessed 5 March 2025

Smith, Graham Hingangaroa, H. and Linda Tuhiwai Smith. 2019. Doing Indigenous work: Decolonizing and transforming the academy. In *Handbook of Indigenous education*, eds. Elizabeth Ann McKinley and Linda Tuhiwai Smith, 1075–110. Singapore, Springer Nature

Workman, Kim, and Tracey McIntosh. 2013. Crime, imprisonment and poverty. In *Inequality: A New Zealand crisis*, ed. Max Rashbrook, 120–133. Wellington: Bridget Williams Books

CHAPTER 6

Listening, Witnessing, and Creative Repair: Towards Justice-Oriented Approaches to Valuing Lived Experience Expertise and Trauma-Informed Co-creative Practice

Poppy de Souza and Rebecca J. Moran

Introduction: Working Creatively With/From Lived Experience

In this chapter, we discuss two creative projects that work with or from lived experience expertise to critically reflect on the process of making, valuing, and 'evaluating'. Focusing on lived experience work raises questions of how 'invisible' outcomes are recognised and valued, and how quiet forms of community connection might be prioritised. We position listening, witnessing, and creative repair as central to a justice-oriented, values-based approach that is sensitive to power and difference, and

P. de Souza (✉) · R. J. Moran
University of New South Wales, Sydney, NSW, Australia
e-mail: poppy.desouza@unsw.edu.au

R. J. Moran
e-mail: rebecca.moran@unsw.edu.au

M. Mullen et al. (eds.), *Artful Evaluation for Creative Health and Wellbeing*, New Directions in Cultural Policy Research,
https://doi.org/10.1007/978-3-032-17063-7_6

oriented towards a politics and practice of 'hearing well' (Stauffer 2015, 74–5). This approach prioritises the value (and values) of slow attention, mutual witnessing, and creative reparation in the wake of trauma and grief while also being attuned to the broader politics of voice within the 'evidence of experience' (Bennett 2022, 7). Most importantly, we each seek to work in ways that minimise harm, do not reproduce harm, and/or ways that seek to repair harm. Our approach is guided by the Principles for Action developed for The Big Anxiety (TBA) mental health and arts festival which include creating 'space for dialogue with those who have been silenced, and on topics where silence is culturally encouraged', and to support opportunities for action by 'amplifying the voices of people with lived experience' (Moran and Bennett n. d.).

Throughout the chapter, we engage with the concept of 'lived experience expertise' (Higgins and Lenette 2024; Gibbs 2022; Moran 2024). The lived experience engagement movement is a collection of social movements, borne out of the disability rights and then the psychiatric survivor movements that demanded better status for those labelled 'mentally ill', 'mad' or 'disordered'. Much progress has been made, and sub-groups continue to argue for different finer points, including those fighting for greater lived experience engagement in service provision, public policy, academia, and government. Higgins and Lenette (2024, 3) argue centring lived experience-led knowledge is an 'emancipatory research approach with disruptive and decolonial potentials'. Where the expertise of people and communities with direct experience of key social justice issues are centred, 'Deep listening, continuous reflection, tenacity and moral courage' (Ibid., 4) is required. More recently, it has extended to the arts and mental health where lived experience of trauma, distress, or injustice is increasingly valued as a critical form of expertise within community-based arts, creativity and wellbeing programmes (Bennett 2022; Australia Council for the Arts, 2023). Prioritising and working creatively with/from lived experience-led knowledge holds the potential to disrupt established hierarchies of knowledge production. When approached through a justice frame and applied to arts-health practices, incorporating lived experience-led expertise both highlights and responds to evaluation frameworks that can devalue or de-prioritise embodied knowledges or which silence or constrain political voice. This can also help shape evaluation practices that better attend to embodied, felt and affective experience, as well as silence and the invisible.

For philosopher Miranda Fricker (2007, 1), there are two intersecting forms of epistemic injustice: testimonial and hermeneutical. Testimonial injustice occurs 'when prejudice causes a hearer to give a deflated level of credibility to a speaker's word'. Hermeneutical injustice is a prior stage of injustice. It occurs 'when a gap in collective interpretive resources puts someone at an unfair disadvantage when it comes to making sense of their social experiences'; that is, injustice related to one's status as a valid 'knower'. Valuing and accounting for lived experience as a form of expertise and knowledge in creative research and evaluation could more explicitly align the work with social justice principles and counter epistemic injustice. For us, working creatively with/from lived experience is an ethical social justice practice.

The arts, particularly community-based, socially engaged arts practices, have long been at the forefront of articulating the lived experience of trauma, injustice, harm, stigma, and marginalisation (Australia Council for the Arts 2023). Creative arts-based approaches to health and wellbeing provide people and communities with alternative ways of understanding and articulating embodied experience (Bennett 2022). This demands an expanded conception of health, in the same way that community-engaged arts practice take place in an 'expanded field' (see Loveless, 2019). As Bennett (2022, 9) writes,

> Rather than limiting inquiry to the role of arts in health, we envision mental health as an expanded field and the emergent creative work that might advance it—an inquiry that is grounded in lived experience, rather than defined by the object of mental health.

In arts, health and wellbeing research and evaluation, there are diverse and contested views about what 'counts' as evidence and whose voices and experiences are counted. On the one hand, there has been increased recognition of the 'evidence of experience' (Bennett 2022) within creative approaches to health and mental wellbeing, what might be called a turn to lived experience (Australia Council for the Arts et al. 2022). Yet, on the other hand, *critical* engagement with lived experience is, we argue, lacking. The turn to working with/from lived experience in arts and health comes with its own set of risks; creative research can be instrumentalised or deployed for institutional ends, limited to surface-level inclusion/participation, or depoliticised (Moran 2024). In this chapter we share our critical approaches, which complicate and deepen our understanding of the politics of working creatively with and from lived experience, while also making clear what is at stake when it comes to engaging diverse communities on their own terms.

As many contributors to this edited collection highlight, the politics and relations of making art with/in communities 'on the margins' extend to the politics of cultural measurement and indicators of value (Belfiore and Bennett 2008; MacDowall et al. 2015). Tensions can arise when credibility (not to mention funding) relies on evaluation frameworks that provide 'proof', 'impact', and 'knowability' (Springgay 2022, 136). Attempts to extract and quantify this 'evidence' must be approached with caution. While lived experience brings distinct forms of meaning and value that contribute new understandings of creative wellbeing—including embodied, affective and felt knowledges—not everything can or should be known or extracted.

In the expanded field of arts and health—where collaborative artistic inquiry is transformed by and through lived experience—the tension between 'evidence' and 'experience' can be both a problem and a creative resource through which new collaborative practices can emerge. While not always achieved, Bennett (2022, 5) argues interdisciplinary work bridging arts and health 'evolves not only new practices but new methods of evaluation'. Similarly, Springgay (2022, 14) suggests:

> Evaluation does not come from institutions (an outside) but is realized internal to the project and in relation to those who cocreated it or participated in it. Further, benefits are not quantifiable but reflect on a project's ethical and political responsibilities.

Working creatively with trauma, grief, and loss has required each of us, in different ways, to reconsider how meaning and value are negotiated within and beyond institutional constraints, and in our own (co)creative research. Following Springgay, we reflect on what counts to each of us and how value might be understood in relation to our respective projects, *Holding Breath* and *Big Grief Big Horror*. Rather than comparative or illustrative examples, we show how they each respond—ethically, aesthetically, and politically—to forms of epistemic injustice and attempt to work in reparative ways that prioritise slow attention, care, and mutual witnessing in the wake of structural harm, stigma, and grief. In each work, we engage with (and from within) communities who have experienced some form of epistemic injustice.

Voice and Positionality

Throughout the chapter we shift between using the third person plural 'we' and the first-person singular 'I'. To help the reader, we use font and formatting to distinguish between our voices:

sans serif text, right justified text for Poppy

sans serif, left justified text for Bec

Below, we briefly situate ourselves and establish our critical and reflexive approach. This challenges the idea that researchers and creative practitioners—whether engaged as 'lived experience' experts or otherwise—are detached or outside of the process of knowledge (and value) creation, or hierarchies of value and voice.

I am a non-Indigenous settler of Anglo and Serani (Eurasian-Malaysian) heritage living as an uninvited guest on Yuggera and Turrbal Lands in Meanjin (Brisbane, Australia). I am a cisgender woman who lives with disability and chronic illness. This positionality locates me in specific relationship to the people I engaged with for *Holding Breath*. My research and practice have focused on questions about the politics of listening in the context of injustice and claims to be heard. I locate my work within a broader commitment to developing anti-colonial and justice-oriented methodologies and am guided by intersectional feminist and de/anti-colonial thinking and practice.

* * *

I am a non-Indigenous settler living and working on unceded Whadjuk Nyoongar boodja (Perth, Western Australia). I am a cisgender woman with disabilities and chronic health issues, and carer responsibilities. I had care responsibilities for two immediate family members who died via a murder-suicide in 2016: it is this grief, horror, and trauma that the short film discussed in this chapter is based on. I have long lived and living experience of receiving 'care' in the mental health system, and it is my early-life experiences in the mental health system, and as a witness/victim in the criminal justice system, that laid the foundations for my career as an academic and activist who frequently focuses on pursuing change in harmful systems—particularly the mental health system. My work centres around, and responds to, complex trauma and epistemic injustice, both of which I also have lived experience of.

In the following sections, Poppy will discuss the first stage of *Holding Breath* (2023–2025), a sound-based community project using voice-note exchanges co-created with other women and non-binary people who live with the debilitating and ongoing impacts of Long COVID. Bec will discuss her single channel video installation *Big Grief, Big Horror* (2022), an intimate work which screened as part of The Big Anxiety festival about what it is like to experience and live beyond a family murder-suicide, inviting multiple publics to witness her story.

Holding Breath (2023–2025)

I developed *Holding Breath* as a collaborative, arts-research and sound-based project to explore collective listening, care, and creative connection across unevenly shared and felt thresholds of experience.[1] The impetus for the project was, in part, my experience of living with Long COVID—a term that emerged through patient self-advocacy and online support groups and is located within a long history of patient-consumer advocacy, disability justice movements and collective activism for recognition—and an intention to collaborate with other sick, disabled and chronically ill folks in the wake of pandemic grief and loss.

I was inspired by disability justice care ethics which prioritises un(der)heard voices and places collective, non-hierarchical care and reciprocity at the heart of justice and social change. Disability justice honours the wisdom of sick, disabled, and chronically ill artists and activists—particularly women, trans and non-binary people of colour—and I have learned much from the creative work and activism of Johanna Hedva, Sins Invalid, Mimi Khúc, Mia Mingus, Akemi Nishida, Leah Lakshmi Piepzna-Samarasinha, Alice Wong, and Julia Rose Bak and Tori Hobbs from the Disability Justice Network. Artist and activist Cassie Thornton's ongoing project *The Hologram*—a 'feminist peer-to-peer health model for a post-pandemic future' which models a distributed network of reciprocal care, support, and solidarity—was also an inspiration.

[1] Ethics Approval: The study was performed in line with the principles of the Declaration of Helsinki. Approval was granted by the Ethics Committee of the University of New South Wales (November 2023/iRECS0816).

While the pandemic transformed our social, cultural, and political landscape, state responses in Australia and beyond exacerbated entrenched health inequities, vulnerabilities, and injustices. Members of the Australian Long COVID Community (ALCC)—an online peer support group of which I am a member—described the experience of living with Long COVID as one of 'epistemic injustice' (Fricker 2007). Grief, frustration, and anger are common emotions for many within the group, along with feelings of not being heard or being dismissed or denied.

Responding to this context, *Holding Breath* invited a handful of women and non-binary people who live with Long COVID and experience 'breathlessness' to take part. The invitation was distributed via online peer support groups and my own networks. My aim was to create space for collective witnessing across shared, *yet distinct*, sites of grief, loss, and debility. An extract from the Briefing Note below sets out what Rajni Shah (2021) calls the 'invitational frame'—the creative container which provided the project's protocols for reciprocal listening and creative exchange:

'In this project, we will make, share, listen and respond to short voice-note memos together. A good way to think about them is like a sound version of hand-written letters. They capture everyday moments. I will record the first voice-note memo and send it to your phone. Listen to it and record a response back to me within a week of receiving it. I will then listen and record a second voice-note memo in response, and so forth until we have exchanged five voice-note memos between us. [...] There are no fixed expectations around what you might want to record. We start with where we're at, with attention to how our bodies and minds, or bodyminds, are feeling. You might record what seems like 'nothing'; if that is all you can do, that is something too. [...] Most importantly, take your time. Go slowly. Breathe'.

Voice-note memos were chosen for the sonic intimacy of the format as well as for accessibility—a creative methodology which invited a mode of encounter that was generative, reciprocal, and often poetic. After an asynchronous exchange of five voice-notes, each collaborator and I came together online in shared temporal space to reflect on the meaning and value of the process. This element was framed as a semi-structured interview for the formal university ethics application, but was, in practice, guided by a reciprocal ethics of care rather than

an evaluation 'add on' and was at the heart of the project's
justice-oriented listening approach.

Like our voice-note memos, our 'interviews' were not conducted to generate 'data' or be extracted as 'evidence' to evaluate. In the first stage, there was no 'public' outcome. Rather, my hope was to find a form that worked to redistribute care and attention in non-hierarchical ways – including by situating myself within the project. While *Holding Breath* prioritised collective care and connection, the creative process was explicitly 'difference attuned' (Rice et al. 2021) such that lines of power and privilege might be gently navigated.

One community collaborator reflected on the intersections of ableism and racism and the ways in which medical negligence disproportionately kills people of colour. Their voice-notes drew attention to the ways hierarchies of power and attention that condition whose voices are heard and valued within broader narratives of health and illness (and within the dynamics of the project itself). While Long COVID was very much on their mind, so was the reporting of an unfolding genocide in Gaza and the debilitating conditions for temporary migrants living with Long COVID.

Sara Ahmed reminds us that 'solidarity does not assume that our struggles are the same struggles, or that our pain is the same pain' (2004, 189). Rather, solidarity involves 'the recognition that even if we do not have the same feelings, or the same lives, or the same bodies, we do live on common ground' (Ibid). Yet what constitutes 'common ground' is always shifting and cannot be assumed. The voice-note methodology provided an intimate space for connection across multiple temporalities and political geographies of debilitation—in ways that afforded solace and solidarity.

Big Grief, Big Horror (2022)

Working creatively with and from lived experience is a cornerstone value informing/guiding how I approach academic and creative work. In my work I am always seeking to find, nurture, fight for, and build spaces where mental distress is responded to in a more human way;

in a way that attends to grief and trauma and is not defined by power imbalances between systems and their users. I am concerned that current mainstream mental health services—which I have recent living experience of—are still not trauma-informed or culturally safe. I started my career as part of the social movement for lived experience regarding mental distress to be given credibility and validity, and I consider this a battle for epistemic justice (Fricker 2007). When I work with my own lived experience, I do so with the knowledge that certain privileges have led to the epistemic justice I usually enjoy: I am someone, my voice can be heard, I am taken as being worth something, and my work is worth something by virtue of the places it is exhibited. With this privilege in mind, I seek to use my voice to the utmost efficacy regarding social injustices, silenced groups, and unspeakable truths. The baring of my lived experience in *Big Grief, Big Horror* was a continuation of my work in this area.

Justice, in my conceptualisation, is always about dignity (Hicks 2011) and recognition (Honneth 1996), which is another way to say 'mattering': you matter, your experience matters, your complaints of harm experienced or of structural injustice matter to your community, and your suffering is meaningful. Judith Herman (2024), in her exploration of what justice means for survivors of trauma and abuse, emphasises the importance of public testimony and shared public outrage as necessary for the reparation of harm, including the epistemic harm commonly experienced by survivors, many of whom have faced disbelief and discreditation. While *Big Grief Big Horror* is a survivor story, it is not the type of trauma story that is commonly undermined, as sexual assault and abuse testimony so often still is (Herman 2024).

In my video artwork *Big Grief Big Horror*, I sit at a table with a cup of tea, talking, sometimes showing emotion, about the murder-suicide of my father and brother at a time in my life when I had a very young baby. I was careful in designing the film to create a sense of intimacy: as if the viewer was sitting on the other side of the table, in conversation with me.[2] I use my multiple positionalities (survivor, scholar, artist, educator) to destabilise notions that people with severe mental distress and a complex history can't also be the lecturer at the

[2] Installation images can be viewed here: https://feel-lab.org/research_projects/big-grief-big-horror/

front of the hall or the researcher who produces empirical and reflexive research outputs. I am in many ways in a 'Goldilocks zone' for public consumption of my lived experience: the distress I show is not too messy, but also not too clean. This was not always true, however, and in my life I have been injured many times, and profoundly, by epistemic injustice. I was a homeless child, a psychiatric patient, a substance user, and a victim of gendered violence and abuse: all positions where I felt the real daily harm of epistemic injustice. My testimony was not credible or valuable. I was further marginalised by this, and suffered deep epistemic harm, with complex trauma messages telling me I could not believe in my own knowledge or capacity to ever be a knower (Fricker 2007).

Of course, justice is a debated and dynamic term, used in many different disciplines as well as in community systems and activities, and in the realm of socially engaged arts and social justice interventions to support community health and wellbeing. But there is a lack of consensus on what it means. There are many 'brands' of justice, including transitional, retributive, restorative, and reparative justice. Different justice frameworks refer to fairness, equity, restoration, a sense of 'right', but also vindication, validation, accountability, punishment, and an array of differently charged core concerns.

In *Big Grief, Big Horror* I was interested in theories of justice and repair in the wake of structural harm and trauma which work towards reconstituting dignity for survivors (Herman 2024; Hicks 2011), and in trauma-informed, anti-oppressive participatory arts practice (Moran and Bennett n.d.; Sunderland et al. 2023).

It does not take much to imagine the grief and horror that I went through, for example, in finding my father's body, but what may be more difficult to imagine is the resilience, humanity, growth, and warmth that also fills the space of this film. My purpose in making the film was to reach out to others who were experiencing unthinkable grief, loss, and trauma, and say 'we can survive this. We can keep going, and even find beauty in our experience.' I wanted to show others with unthinkable traumas that we can survive annihilation; that we can (but don't have to) thrive and be creative in the midst of it; that we are not stalled as people while deep in grief but are still part of the community—still alive.

I was the 'participant' and the 'lived experience expert', but also director and designer (with my remote team located across Australia). This is of value to me, as I had agency and control over what my video testimony would be; an experience of particular importance considering my previous experiences of epistemic injustice. I purposefully spoke with raw openness and honesty about my big grief and big horror, with the belief that surviving the extreme edges of human experiences might have taught me something of value to share.

I also included moments of lightness and humour, and spoke of the love and aesthetic acuity I experienced after my father and brother's deaths. In preparing and delivering this unscripted monologue to camera, I built a picture in my mind of who I was talking to. In particular, I wanted to reach out to anyone who might be suffering in a similar way, as I felt they might find value in relating to me. Big grief and big horror make one alien; we are frozen in time while, for other people, the sun keeps coming up and going down, and 'Monday' remains an important construct. Immense grief can stay unspoken, not least for fear of causing discomfort or contagion, leaving the grieving effectively silenced and isolated: further epistemic injustice. The deployment of lived experience, and speaking the unspeakable, is an act of resistance in a world where the mad have for centuries been discredited and dismissed.

I hoped that my film would reach out a hand to those falling in the void, and from all feedback received, it worked. For the duration of The Big Anxiety festival where the film was shown on demand in a gallery space with another Big Anxiety film installation. I was frequently approached by people wanting to thank me for the film and telling me how valuable it had been for them to sit with me and hear this story of annihilation and resilience. This gave me yet another position of engagement with the process of making and sharing the creative work—my being present, live, and available to approach and talk to during the screenings gave people an opportunity to take their connection with me further—by telling me of their griefs, or just that they had griefs. Exhibited in a quiet space, alongside work that also invited quiet reflection, the work became reciprocal and levelling. This kind of value is difficult to measure or capture an impression of, but I cannot ignore the compelling sense of value as I hug and cry with someone who tells me their life has been changed by seeing this short film, a story of human survival, loss and love.

Listening, Witnessing, and Creative Repair

Holding Breath and *Big Grief, Big Horror* each work creatively with experiences of grief, trauma, and loss to generate registers of mediated testimony—narrative, poetic—that are heard and witnessed by specific intimate publics across different thresholds of experience. While we don't want to overwhelm readers with theory, we do feel it is important to include and briefly cite some of the key thinkers who have informed our understandings of listening, witnessing and repair, and which are relevant to the works we discuss in the chapter. To us, they are central to our argument regarding evaluation of justice-oriented arts, health and wellbeing practice that engages with lived experience.

Jill Stauffer (2015), writing in the context of institutional and structural harm, terms the injustice of not being heard as 'ethical loneliness'. In the wake of trauma, loss, 'big grief' (Moran 2022), or epistemic injustice (Fricker 2007), there is much at stake in working creatively with/from lived experience and care must be taken. Both forms of injustice speak to the conditions of credibility, the politics of knowledge and questions of justice and power; of whose experiences are heard, believed, valued, and witnessed, and the terms through which differently positioned groups can give account of the conditions of their lives. The creative mode of testimonial practice of *Big Grief, Big Horror*, for example, works against ethical loneliness to prioritise survivor-led meaning making and value. It transforms an individual, private experience of living in the wake of profound family trauma, grief, and loss by inviting an intimate public to bear witness within a broader ecology of social relations and anchored in a feminist ethics of reception. In *Holding Breath,* the intention was to build a relational project that was 'attentive' rather than 'declarative' (Shah 2021, 47)—offering a register of testimony that was gentle, tender, and which afforded space for poetic response and reciprocity.

The 'turn to listening' has gained increasing currency in several fields—in arts, health, and social policy. Yet listening is neither universal nor neutral and is fraught with tension. Stauffer (2015, 74–5) insists that 'hearing well' is not about smooth or easy listening—listening not as a route to empathy or a moral cure—but a justice-oriented and political practice. For us, political listening is located within a broader concern for ethical relations and responsibility in the context of difference, injustice, and inequality. The transformative potential for listening and witnessing lies not (or not only) in shifts in individual emotional terrains, but in the broader conditions and relations which shape collective possibilities for being heard. To hear well, following Stauffer, requires an openness to listen across difference (Dreher 2009), in ways that might be uncomfortable, (de Souza and Dreher 2021), and yet open to tenderness (McDowell 2022).

The ethics of witnessing was another consideration in each of our projects. Carla Rice and colleagues (2021) draw on feminist, Black, Indigenous, and affect theories to develop the notion of 'difference-attuned witnessing' to account for social inequities and asymmetries in power in the co-design of processes of creative engagement with diverse communities. Difference-attuned witnessing suggests a mode of ethical responsiveness that moves beyond empathy, where over-identification can collapse (or consume) difference; yet neither does it suggest a dispassionate observer of distant suffering. Rather, it suggests a felt and proximate politics of witnessing. This chimes with Kelly Oliver's (2015, 475) formulation of witnessing, grounded in response ethics, which requires a move *beyond* identification and recognition to embrace 'the affective and imaginative dimensions of experience'. Both *Holding Breath* and *Big Horror, Big Grief* designed-in opportunities for ethical listening and witnessing to occur between specific and differently located communities of collaborators or intimate publics.

Naomi Toth and Lily Hibberd (2021, 94) use the term 'creative reparation' to describe alternative modes of creative testimony and voice aimed at mending the harms of individual and collective trauma or grief. They write about the immersive video work *Parragirls Past, Present* (2019) made in collaboration with Parragirls—survivors of debilitating gendered violence and abuse and state-sanctioned harm while teenagers at the former Paramatta Girls Home in Sydney. Despite the impossibilities of repair, Parragirls found small and mighty ways to survive and forged creative connections in the wake of their experience. *Parragirls Past, Present* emerged from an impulse that sought to restore dignity through creative practice grounded in collective care, beyond institutional models of state reparations (see Hibberd and Djuric 2019).

A reparative thread can be traced through the process of co/creating *Big Grief, Big Horror* and *Holding Breath* in as much as each work sought to create spaces of connection, solace and solidarity through creative expression (for us and the intimate publics we engaged with) in ways that did not reproduce harm, and which held the potential for transformation and social repair. Importantly, the meaning and value of these projects were not contingent on, nor evaluated by, extractive metrics of impact external to each work. This distinction reveals an essential point about the theory discussed in this chapter: that meaning and value are not to be extracted from creative projects to serve an external or instrumental purpose. Rather, they are integral to the practice itself, grounded in the same critical and artistic principles and ideas that shape the work. This approach underscores the importance of understanding evaluation not as something imposed from outside, but as an inherent component of a justice-oriented approach—one that arises organically from the project's own ethical and artistic intentions, while honouring the expertise that comes with lived experience.

Towards a Justice-Oriented Approach

If being heard can repair ethical loneliness,
if we translate Jill Stauffer,
then to be witnessed amongst the wreckage
is a reminder that selves and worlds are
made, remade and undone -
always in relation
and always in relations of power.

So, mattering
means dignity
which,
if we translate Judith Herman
means justice.

We close by highlighting connections and distinctions across our processes of creative engagement with community that emerged from conversations and exchanges between us during our writing of this chapter. In one of our conversations on Zoom, as we were trying to follow the many threads and concepts we've charted across the chapter—each of us in affective states of exhaustion and vulnerability and moving at a snail's pace—we found our orientation: *witnessing means mattering means dignity means justice*. Our concerns, we reflected, were informed by the need to respond creatively to forms of epistemic injustice in reparative ways that centre those who have been harmed or unheard, and/

or work in ways that don't reproduce harm or ways that seek to repair harm. The poetic fragments above were exchanged in an email thread and helped us to ground theory in lived experience—to critically reflect on the world 'as it is given to us' (Ahmed 2023, 128, italics in original). In this process, we came to see how each of us shares a values-led approach to co-creative practice and community engagement that prioritises and works in company with lived experience expertise. Ethical considerations around the politics of listening, witnessing, and creative repair guide each of us to move slowly and with attention to our own positionalities and investments in the work that we do.

We do not speak from the same position
or with one voice
our margins are drawn across intersecting lines
We each carry histories and stories that may never be shared
We are not generalisable,
some of us are incomprehensible
We are not always yours to know.
But yes, we are weary, this is true.
Not in the same way,
and not with the same stakes.
it is our relation of approach that matters

We are not the Neoliberalists' Dream.
And yes, you should be worried,
because we know how to connect
We know how to ***be*** with such value
that our revolution is seeded despite our weariness

Each of our projects were designed with different, if intersecting, frameworks of justice in mind (disability justice, epistemic justice) and our work is in conversation with scholarship, activism and practice that spans diverse disciplines and histories. What we offer in this chapter is an orientation towards justice to foreground and situate any reflection on the meaning, value and significance of participatory or relational arts projects within the specific histories, entanglements and relations of power from which they emerge. We aim to move beyond traditional evaluation frameworks, which can be instrumentalised or used to promote or focus on individual responsibility for change. Instead, we propose an approach for engaging with lived experience work and community-engaged creative practice, prioritising the value (and values) of slow attention, mutual witnessing, and creative reparation in the wake of structural harm, stigma, and grief while also being attuned to the broader politics of voice within the 'evidence of experience' (Bennett 2022). We have come to value listening, witnessing, and repair as practical and political resources which can be harnessed creatively and inform a values-based approach that gets to the heart of our community-engaged arts-research practices.

References

Ahmed, Sara. 2004. *The cultural politics of emotion*. Second edition. Edinburgh: Edinburgh University Press.

Ahmed. 2023. *The Feminst Killjoy Handbook: The Radical Potential of Getting in the Way*. Penguin Press.

Australia Council for the Arts, Jill Bennett, Katherine Boydell, Jane Davidson, and Claire Hooker. 2022. *Arts, creativity and mental wellbeing: Research, practice and lived experience*. Discussion Paper. Sydney: Australia Council for the Arts. https://creative.gov.au/wp-content/uploads/2022/04/Creativity-and-Wellbeing-Summit-Discussion-Paper-updated.pdf

Australia Council for the Arts. 2023. *Connected Lives: Creative solutions to the mental health crisis*. Sydney: Australia Council for the Arts. https://creative.gov.au/wp-content/uploads/2023/02/Connected-Lives-Creative-solutions-to-the-mental-health-crisis-Web-version.pdf

Belfiore, Elanora and Oliver Bennett. 2008. *The social impact of the arts*. Hampshire: Palgrave Macmillan

Bennett, Jill. 2022. The politics of experience and the function of art in the expanded field of mental health. In *The Big Anxiety: Taking care of mental health in times of crisis*, ed. Jill Bennett, 3–14. London: Bloomsbury

de Souza, Poppy, and Tanja Dreher. 2021. Dwelling in discomfort: On the conditions of listening in settler ial Australia. *Borderlands Journal* 20(2): 30–60. https://doi.org/10.21307/borderlands-2021-012

Dreher, Tanja. 2009 Listening Across Difference: Media and multiculturalism beyond the politics of voice. *Continuum*, 23(4): 445–458, https://doi.org/10.1080/10304310903015712

Fricker, Miranda. 2007. *Epistemic injustice: Power and the ethics of knowing*. Oxford: Oxford University Press.

Gibbs, El. 2022. Lived expertise means experts. http://elgibbs.com.au/lived-expertise-means-experts/. Accessed 30 January 2024.

Herman, Judith. 2024. *Truth and repair: How trauma survivors envision justice*. London: Hachette.

Hibberd, Lily, and Bonney Djuric. 2019. *Parragirls*: Reimagining Parramatta Girls Home through art and memory. Sydney: New South Books.

Hicks, Donna. 2011. *Dignity: The essential role it plays in resolving conflict*. New Haven: Yale University Press.

Hibberd, Lily, and Bonney Djuri. 2019. *Parragirls: Reimagining Parramatta Girls Home Through Art and Memory*. Sydney, NSW: New South Books.

Higgins, Maree, and Caroline Lenette. 2024. *Disrupting the academy with lived experience-led knowledge*. London: Policy Press.

Honneth, Axel. 1996. *The struggle for recognition: the moral grammar of social conflicts*. Cambridge: MIT press.

Loveless, Natalie. 2019. *How to make art at the end of the world: A manifesto for research-creation* Durham: Duke University Press.

MacDowall, Lachlan, Marnie Badham, Emma Blomkamp, and Kim Dunphy. (eds). 2015. *Making culture count: The politics of cultural measurement*. London: Palgrave Macmillan.

McDowell, Amanda. 2022. Hold me in a circle of tender listening: Entangled encounters with women survivors from the Mental Health Testimony Project archive. In *The Big Anxiety: Taking care of mental health in times of crisis*, ed. Jill Bennett, 223–236. London: Bloomsbury.

Moran, Rebecca J. 2022. *Big Grief, Big Horror. Medium: Single channel video*. The Big Anxiety festival.

Moran, Rebecca J. 2024. Towards a scholarship of critical lived experience engagement: Big feelings, big stories, big learning. In *Disrupting the academy with lived experience-led knowledge*, eds. Maree Higgins and Caroline Lenette. 36–50. Bristol: Polity Press.

Moran Rebecca J. and Jill Bennett. n.d. *The Big Anxiety*'s Principles for Action https://www.thebiganxiety.org/about/.

Oliver, Kelly. 2015. Witnessing, recognition, and response ethics. *Philosophy & Rhetoric* 48(4): 473–93. https://doi.org/10.5325/philrhet.48.4.0473

Rice, Carla, Katie Cook, and K Alysse Bailey. 2021. Difference-attuned witnessing: Risks and potentialities of arts-based research. *Feminism & Psychology* 3(3): 345–65. https://doi.org/10.1177/0959353520955142.

Shah, Rajni. 2021. *Experiments in listening*. London: Rowman & Littlefield.

Springgay, Stephanie. 2022. *Feltness: Research-creation, socially engaged art, and affective pedagogies*. Durham, NC: Duke University Press.

Stauffer, Jill. 2015. *Ethical loneliness: The injustice of not being heard*. New York: Columbia University Press.

Sunderland, Naomi, Fiona Stevens, Kate Knudsen, Rae Cooper, and Marianne Wobcke. 2023. Trauma aware and anti-oppressive arts-health and community arts practice: Guiding principles for facilitating healing, health and wellbeing. *Trauma, Violence, & Abuse* 24(4): 2429–47. https://doi.org/10.1177/15248380221097442.

Toth, Naomi, and Lily Hibberd. 2021. *Parragirls Past, Present: Unlocking Memories of Institutional 'Care'*: Witnessing and Creative Reparation in the Aftermath of Parramatta Girls Home. *Synthesis: An Anglophone Journal of Comparative Literary Studies* 13(July): 94–114. https://doi.org/10.12681/syn.27563.

PART III

Community Wellbeing, Participation and Self-Determination

CHAPTER 7

Experimenting with Life in Vacant Spaces: Reflections on Assessing and Communicating Holistic Wellbeing Outcomes

Kelly Dombroski

Introduction

Measuring and communicating the holistic value of community wellbeing initiatives is a fraught task. On the one hand, the very nature of holistic initiatives means that interdependent and interacting factors cannot easily be connected to specific outcomes. On the other hand, if there is not some form of measurement and accounting, the ongoing sustainability of the initiatives can be called into question—are they actually doing anything worthwhile? Is it worth continuing to invest time, money, and energy into these initiatives? These are questions that I have been asking over several different projects with various colleagues, resulting in a few different answers including qualitative assessments (Dombroski et al.

K. Dombroski (✉)
Massey University, Palmerston North, New Zealand
e-mail: K.Dombroski@massey.ac.nz

Te Aparangi Royal Society, Wellington, New Zealand

M. Mullen et al. (eds.), *Artful Evaluation for Creative Health and Wellbeing*, New Directions in Cultural Policy Research,
https://doi.org/10.1007/978-3-032-17063-7_7

2018, 2019; Healy et al. 2019), social return on investment-style analyses with dollar figures (Clare et al. 2023), a few unpublished attempts at working through a quantitative methodology of a Community Economy Return on investment (Gibson-Graham et al. 2013; Petrescu et al. 2021) and indicator-based community systems of assessment and planning for wellbeing (Yates et al. 2023).

My inquiry into evaluation methods began in 2014 as an early career researcher with training in community economies and development studies, when Irene Boles took me out for coffee. I had recently begun working at the University of Canterbury in Ōtautahi Christchurch as a lecturer, and was casting around for projects I could do in the resource-constrained post-earthquake environment with little funding and limited travel due to small children. Irene was an educator and researcher at Ara Polytechnic and the chairperson of the board of the charitable trust Life in Vacant Spaces (LiVS). She told me that Life in Vacant Spaces had started in response to the mass demolitions in central Christchurch after the devastating earthquakes in Canterbury in 2010 and 2011. The organisation brokered vacant land for temporary use projects for artists and other educational or entrepreneurial projects. She had noted on my university profile that I was interested in community economies and community-led action research. She came to me to ask if I could help her out with calculating the value of the work conducted by the post-quake organisation she was involved with (see Box 1).

Box 1: Life in Vacant Spaces

Life in Vacant Spaces (LiVS) is a charitable trust in Ōtautahi, Christchurch that brokers spaces for community groups, creative projects, social enterprises, and start-ups to undertake (primarily) transitional activities. The organisation connects owners of vacant land and buildings with people who have ideas to fill those spaces, usually temporarily. LiVS provides support from the initial stages of ideas and brainstorming, through to deinstallation. This support includes providing:

- agreements or insurance to reduce the risk to the project for all involved
- social connections and support (including mentors and sponsors)
- key infrastructure or basic upgrades to ensure appropriate spaces for a range of projects
- advice on project management, funding, and event support.

At the time of research, LiVS employed two part-time staff, a director and a project manager, had occasional contractors, and relied on staff using their own communication and transport assets. The organisation rented some desks in a co-working space at a previous LiVS supported project. For most of its history, the organisation had to apply for funding every year. In 2021, for the first time, the organisation was given three years of funding by Christchurch City Council. The charitable trust is governed by a board of trustees.

LiVS started in 2012, soon after the Canterbury earthquake sequences of 2010 and 2011. These earthquakes devastated the city and its residents, with vast swathes of the central city becoming vacant space. Yet, what emerged from this vacant space and the struggles of recovery was a desire for creativity and change. In many ways this enabled new possibilities as the city and its residents recovered from the physical and psychological impacts. The organisation was formed after a report commissioned by Christchurch City Council (CCC) and written by Gap Filler founders Ryan Reynolds and Coralie Winn. Since then, over 700 projects and numerous organisations have been enabled through LiVS support.

By providing spaces for community-led projects, LiVS has enabled a diverse range of initiatives that contribute to the city's recovery and resilience. The earthquakes not only caused extensive physical damage but also disrupted the social fabric of the community. In this context, it was not necessarily entrepreneurial and physical rebuild initiatives, but *arts* initiatives that emerged as a powerful means of supporting wellbeing and fostering a sense of community. Public art installations, creative workshops, and community-driven exhibitions have played a significant role in the healing process, offering residents a way to express their experiences and rebuild their lives (Cloke and Conradson 2018; Cloke et al. 2023). Each year, Irene told me, LiVS prepares a report detailing some of their outcomes, but like many charitable trusts, had struggled to communicate the value of their work in terms that made sense to funders and others unfamiliar with the wellbeing outcomes of transitional place-making.

In their reporting, LiVS could count things, like the number of projects enabled, or the square metres of project space in temporary lease situations, or the number of inquiries converted into projects. However, Irene felt that these things had limited meaning without the wider context. She wanted to know if I could convert all this into a dollar value somehow, including multiplier effects and so on. At that point, I had heard of such methods, but I had no ability to do that kind of work. In fact, I felt that my work to recognise holistic wellbeing outcomes in community development were often directly opposed to such methods, which tend to partition off certain effects from the whole, and to encourage a mindset of organisational and project growth. Instead, I preferred a community development approach, where success is often defined as when the organisation is no longer needed. Yet, I was fascinated with the work LiVS were doing and could immediately see how it was a form of collectivising responsibility for wellbeing in a city where community action was often happening more quickly than central or local government could respond. I first collaborated with Irene on an article about the value of the transitional commoning LiVS was enabling (Dombroski et al. 2019), but the question of how to measure and communicate value holistically stayed with me. Over the next decade, this question guided me as I put together different teams and sought funding to answer it. This book chapter is one attempt at making sense of my efforts to answer this question.

The chapter proceeds as follows. First, I introduce a range of LiVS-enabled initiatives to give the reader a sense of what we were trying to assess. I then outline the methods I used in collaboration with LiVS employees to select and document a range of initiatives. I then introduce the holistic assessment tools I assembled to help with assessing wellbeing in particular. In the last section, I summarise the wellbeing outcomes and demonstrate the efficacy of the particular method of participatory evaluation used with reference to the arts. I conclude with some thoughts about assessing wellbeing holistically and what the next steps might be in this journey of communicating the holistic value of arts as community work.

Initiatives Enabled by Life in Vacant Spaces

LiVS supports art installations, studios and events, community groups, start-up businesses, and environmental projects. The projects should contribute to educational, cultural, environmental, or entrepreneurial goals and are assessed by the project manager in terms of need, uniqueness, accessibility, planning and finance, experience, and the kind of space required. After the ideas proposed are checked against the criteria, LiVS might offer support to develop the ideas, a referral, or a commitment to help broker a space for the project. LiVS works with the individual or organisation to find a space, negotiate with the landowner to get access, develop and use a simple participation agreement with flexible rolling term, help arrange insurance and consents, and provide practical support as needed (see Box 2).

Box 2: Examples of projects that LiVs has enabled

What kinds of projects has LiVS enabled in Ōtautahi Christchurch? It has:

- provided and managed space in an abandoned school for a community of artists, including Free Theatre, Christchurch's long running avantgarde theatre society.
- provided space for Christchurch Aunties to store furniture and everyday supplies for women's refuges and their clients.
- brokered land for Cultivate Christchurch, who integrates youth employment training and organic urban farming to support youth wellbeing.
- brokered indoor and outdoor spaces for The Green Lab, which focuses on urban greening and community connection through temporary landscaping projects.
- supported a young person to start a gelato business in a caravan on temporary-lease land, which is now a chain of gelato shops.
- supported the New Brighton community to self-manage Roy Stokes Hall for a variety of community projects including circus training, playgroups, and events.
- partnered with Gap Filler, who uses temporary space to create temporary urban projects to foster community engagement and creativity.
- supported Watch This Space to get permissions for urban art projects and exhibitions to enhance public spaces.
- subsidised spaces at Salt Lane Studios, a workspace for artists and creatives to collaborate.
- managed East x East, transforming vacant earthquake damaged land into community spaces for various projects and activities, including Redzone Drone Racing, an all-ages club for building and racing drones, and Disc Golf at East x East.

It is immediately clear from this small proportion represented in Box 2 that the diversity of projects is quite significant—and any single measure of success is not suitable. I worked with the LiVS board (of which I became a member) and the staff to develop a project that would help assess the holistic wellbeing outcomes of these widely divergent projects.

Developing Methods Together

With colleagues, I initially got funding to work with one LiVS-enabled project, Cultivate Christchurch, to co-develop an assessment tool and rubric for evaluating and communicating their wellbeing outcomes for youth, environment, and wider community. We developed an intensive workshop-based method for co-designing a rubric with an NGO (Dombroski et al. 2018). In 2020, then director Rachel Shiels got some funding from the George Sevicke Jones Trust to conduct research into the wellbeing effects of their work on the East x East space. East x East is a nine-hectare space in the east of Ōtautahi Christchurch, where hundreds of houses had been demolished following the 2010 and 2011 earthquakes. Between 2019 and 2022, LiVS employed Burwood resident Hannah Watkinson to set up transitional and long-term projects in the site, with community partners in this lower-income suburb. It quickly became clear that the intensive method developed with Cultivate would not be suitable for assessing the hundreds of wide-ranging projects that LiVS had enabled.

To kick us off with developing our methods, I held a workshop in 2021 with the LiVS board and staff. The group decided that an exhibition, book, and report would meet the needs of both LiVS and the researchers.[1] The group brainstormed projects and organisations that LiVS had supported that would demonstrate the *range* of activities rather than the *most common* activities. From a list of potential projects developed by (then) LiVS director Rachael Shiels and reviewed by the board, we approached 34 people to be interviewed. Of these, I was able to interview thirteen in 2021. Some of these interviews covered more than one project/organisation, because the interviewee had been involved with more than one. Participants also provided the research team with relevant documents about their projects and organisation (including independent and internal reports), and reviewed their own transcripts. I also reviewed publicly available information about other LiVS-supported projects and organisations. Altogether, 27 projects/organisations were reviewed as part of the research, 12 of which were arts-related.

[1] Social research ethics for the project was obtained through Manaaki Whenua—Landcare Research.

Following this, I analysed the transcripts, associated documents supplied by participants, and publicly available material using a qualitative coding method in NVivo, a software programme that helps organise and code qualitative material for themes. We used two sets of codes, inductive (emerging from the material) and deductive (researcher-driven). The inductive codes helped identify facts about the organisations, the concerns, values, and understandings of the interviewees. They included 'volunteers', 'funding', and 'COVID-19', for example. The deductive codes helped us to connect the material to wider urban wellbeing literature and also organise for our exhibition. They included 'mission', 'connection', and 'place', which helped us connect the wellbeing outcomes with themes in international and national wellbeing research.

The coded transcripts were then used to construct the analysis matrix. This matrix included a brief description of the project/organisation, key quotes that exemplified their relationship with LiVS or their contribution to the wellbeing of the city, and an assessment of the projects/organisations impacts and returns according to the following wellbeing frameworks in Box 3. We were highly attuned to the fact that we were conducting this research in a settler-colonial country on Indigenous land. As such, we were keen to create space for frameworks that enabled Māori worldviews and wellbeing values to be part of the analysis, selecting frameworks developed from Māori worldviews by Māori researchers that had been released for general use in Aotearoa New Zealand.

Box 3: Wellbeing frameworks used in analysis matrix

1. Sustainable Development Goals
2. Te Pae Mahutonga public health framework (Durie 1999)
3. Community economies ethical coordinates with reference to the Community Economy Return on Investment (CEROI) concept (J. K. Gibson-Graham, Cameron, and Healy 2013)
4. Mauri Ora/living systems compass tool (Yates 2021)

We also trialled mapping the contributions against the Five Ways to Wellbeing framework[2] but found it did not suit the work of LiVS because this framework is mainly about individual actions for wellbeing rather than

[2] See, https://mentalhealth.org.nz/five-ways-to-wellbeing.

wider community and city-scale actions. While many LiVS projects create space for individuals to act for their wellbeing, they extend beyond this to collective actions. Collective approaches to wellbeing are important for long term sustainability and for justice between groups with different access to individual resources (Kamp et al. 2022).

We tested the draft analysis matrix with the interview case studies and reviewed it with the exhibition project team led by LiVS[3] to see how the different frameworks resonated with their vision for the exhibition. The project action team chose to use the CEROI and Mauri Ora frameworks for analysis because the CEROI foregrounded important ethical questions and intentions, and the Mauri Ora Compass tool enabled different kinds of wellbeing outcomes to be communicated. In addition to this, the project partners were keen to practice reciprocity by engaging with the tools and frameworks that the wider research team had been involved in developing.[4]

Assessment Tools

People and organisations supported by LiVS intentionally invest time and energy into activities and projects hoping for a certain return or outcome. In many of these initiatives, the hoped-for outcome was some form of urban activity or activation. For Ōtautahi Christchurch, urban activations sought to create vibrancy in an otherwise tragic environment recovering from a sequence of earthquakes. This was the case in many of the LiVS-supported central city and East x East projects, which focused on activating areas that had been vacated because of earthquake-related effects, such as liquefaction, building demolitions, or damage. However, urban activations can also be about place-making—creating environments that reflect the values, desires, and stories of the people who live there. Sometimes urban activations might be experimental trials of architecture, art, or community development practices that invite residents to think about and even imagine their place differently. But how to explain the

[3] The project action team included: Rachael Shiels (LiVS director from 2018 to 2021), Hannah Watkinson (coordinator of the LiVS managed East x East space from 2018 to 2021), Elisha Blogg (LiVS director from 2021), and Kelly Dombroski (lead researcher).

[4] This part of the research was funded by Building Better Homes, Towns, and Cities Urban Wellbeing workstream. Principal Investigator was Associate Professor Amanda Yates.

holistic intentions and experimental outcomes of such 'investments' by LiVS?

Community Economy Return on Investment (CEROI)

The Community Economy Return on investment (CEROI) is a method to think about investment in different kinds of economic, social, and ecological futures. Sometimes businesses will have to show how they make decisions based on whether the financial return on investment will be a sum of money larger than the money invested through the use of a 'return on investment'[5] figure using a calculation like the following:

$$\text{ROI} = \frac{(\text{gain from investment} - \text{cost of investment})}{\text{cost of investment}}$$

The CEROI invites users to consider a diverse range of investments, including time and energy as well as money, and a diverse range of returns—including returns in environmental wellbeing and social connection (see Fig. 7.1). This is not a new concept, and many people make decisions like this all the time. However, the CEROI brings visibility to the kinds of investment decisions and intentions people and organisations make when they prioritise other kinds of returns alongside—or in contrast to—only financial returns.

The CEROI was developed by community economies researchers JK Gibson-Graham, Jenny Cameron, and Stephen Healy. In their book *Take Back the Economy* (J. K. Gibson-Graham, Cameron, and Healy 2013), they developed a set of questions to highlight the kinds of economies many people around the world want, where both people and planet can survive well. Rather than providing a strict definition of such an economy, they use six questions to encourage people to consider what such an economy might look like where they live:

- How do we survive together well and equitably?

[5] ROI's main appeal is that it is easy to calculate and has a clear number, but as our collaborator Matthew Scobie points out, it fails to properly account for 'opportunity cost', e.g. what could have been done with the investment otherwise, and 'discounting', e.g. what the future returns on the present investment are calculated to be. We narrated intentions and outcomes from investing for future generations, but we didn't apply a 'discount'. This is aspect of the CEROI that could be further developed in future research.

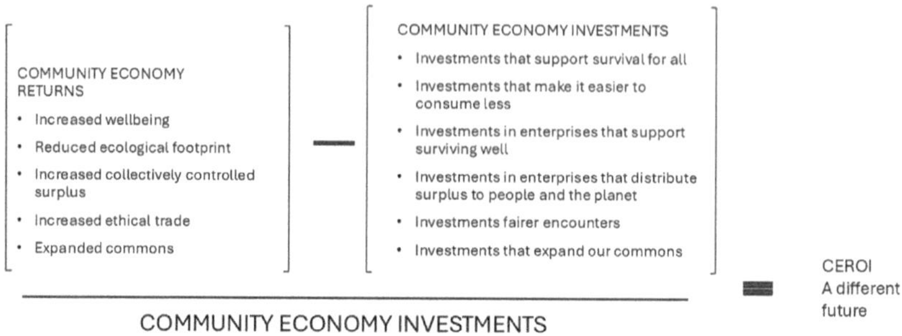

Fig. 7.1 Community Economy Return on investment (Gibson-Graham et al., 2013)

- How do consume sustainably?
- How do we encounter others in ways that support mutual wellbeing?
- How do we distribute surplus and enrich social and environmental health?
- How do we care for the commons that sustain us all?
- How do we invest in future generations? (J. K. Gibson-Graham, Cameron, and Healy 2013).

The authors develop each of these questions in detail, showing a diverse range of ways that people and organisations all over the world have created economic practices where both people and planet can survive together well. In their 2013 book, they proposed the CEROI as a simple way of exploring investments in these kinds of economies.

Undertaking a CEROI is complex, and there have been different approaches to using the method, both qualitative (Dombroski et al. 2019) and quantitative (Petrescu et al. 2021) We could not access the kind of data for each LiVS-supported project that was used for the Cultivate Christchurch or R-Urban examples (given there have been more than 700 individual projects, many of which have finished up and gone on to new iterations). Instead, I used the CEROI approach (and associated six questions) to discuss with participants the kinds of investment intentions and decisions they made, and the kinds of outcomes they observed on these investments. Given I was not attempting to quantify the returns on investment in dollar terms, the approach of analysing self-reported investments, intentions, and outcomes was appropriate (see further discussion in Dombroski et al. 2023).

The intentions of the projects were categorised according to the following core questions taken from the CEROI framework summarised in Box 4.

Box 4: Analysing project intentions using a Community Economies Return on Investment Framework

Surviving well: Investments that support surviving well for all—including psychological needs, beauty, and joy. Because this category is so broad, we focused on the 'well' aspect of surviving well, which is a little different from how Gibson-Graham et al. imagine it in Fig. 7.1. In the analysis, I looked in the transcripts for aspects of psychological release, mental health interventions, connecting with nature and place, and joyful play.

Caring for commons: Investments that expand our commons—so a community of people can be formed around it. Here I looked for evidence that initiatives were sharing resources and spaces with groups of others. It did not have to be completely public, although many of them were, but it did have to have some element of taking something that was privately owned and putting it into community or group use.

Encountering others: Investments in transformative and supportive encounters—where people come to think about others' needs as well as their own. I looked for evidence of initiatives seeking to produce spaces of in-person or distant encounters with others, including animal others.

Rethinking consumption and distribution of surplus: Investments that make it easier to consume less or distribute surplus differently—including planned reductions in consumption, shifting patterns of consumption to support sustainability, and the distribution of surplus to support sustainability. I looked for provocative initiatives that challenged people's consumption, reuse and repair initiatives that changed consumption patterns and also initiatives where people's surplus time and labour were taken up with things that supported others or their own wellbeing.

Investing in futures: Investments in enterprises that distribute surplus to people and planet—including in initiatives that seek to change the world somehow. Here, I examined the transcripts for examples of 'more-than-financial' investment—where some kind of surplus was created, 'saved', and distributed in transformative ways.

Measuring the outcomes of these investments was not simple. Using the same categories to then measure outcomes would also run the risk of losing the holistic outcomes of different investments. One strategy would have been to create indicators to allow someone to measure the extent to which we could see each of these investments making a difference. But another strategy was to juxtapose a holistic wellbeing approach over the matrix and use a multi-faceted communication tool to see what would emerge. This was the choice that the exhibition project team made when deciding how to communicate the outcomes. We contacted Amanda Yates (Ngāti Rangiwewehi, Ngāti Whakaue, Te Aitanga a Māhaki, Rongowhakaata) to collaborate further with her in using the Mauri Ora Compass (Yates, Dombroski, and Dionisio 2023).

Mauri Ora Compass

Rooted in Indigenous Māori perspectives, the Mauri Ora Compass tool effectively created a wellbeing framework, using visual measures of different aspects of wellbeing across multiple dimensions. It provided a holistic view of how projects contribute to the overall vitality of individuals and communities.

The Mauri Ora Compass is intended for use in urban wellbeing transformations, and was developed by Amanda Yates. It has had other iterations since the time we used it for our exhibition and booklet, with different words used and some categories combined or separated out visually.

We described it as follows in the report:

> The Mauri Ora Compass draws on the concept of mauri, understood as the life force inherent in all. It goes beyond Western understandings of animate and inanimate, and foregrounds the life force of rivers, ecosystems, mountains, rocks or buildings alongside that of humans, animals, microbes, plants and more. These things can be in a state of mauri ora (holistic wellbeing), mauri noho (stasis) or mauri mate (decline and illness). The Mauri Ora Compass can help identify how an urban place might navigate towards mauri ora and away from mauri mate. It can also be used to assess how well holistic urban wellbeing outcomes are being achieved. (Dombroski et al. 2023)

The version of the compass we used considers six areas of mauri ora, each extending the word 'ora' which means 'well' in a holistic way. In Yate's formulations, each of these six areas has a list of possible actions that could contribute towards holistic wellbeing in a specific place. We did not use the actions of the Mauri Ora Compass in developing the assessment approach, as we were retrospectively evaluating the kinds of wellbeing outcomes that had occurred from the different activities LiVS had supported. Instead, we understood these as broad areas of wellbeing consideration. We further simplified the action areas into an indicator diagram, highlighting which area/s of the compass the intention and outcome related to (Fig. 7.2).

With consultation with the LiVS project team and Amanda Yates, I set to work categorising the projects according to the following criteria. The bolded titles indicate Amanda's translations for each aspect at the time (Dombroski et al. 2022)—some of which have changed with later versions of the compass (Yates 2022).

Hapori ora—Connected Communities. I categorised the organisation/project as returning hapori ora if it resulted in connecting people together in some way—whether through an event such as performance, or through longer term relationships such as a community garden or sport club. For example, many of GapFiller's projects involved play-based activities in the city, such as a giant video game and the Dance-o-Mat (Fig. 7.3). While a community is generally understood to be a group of people with long-term overlapping geographic or other interests or attributes

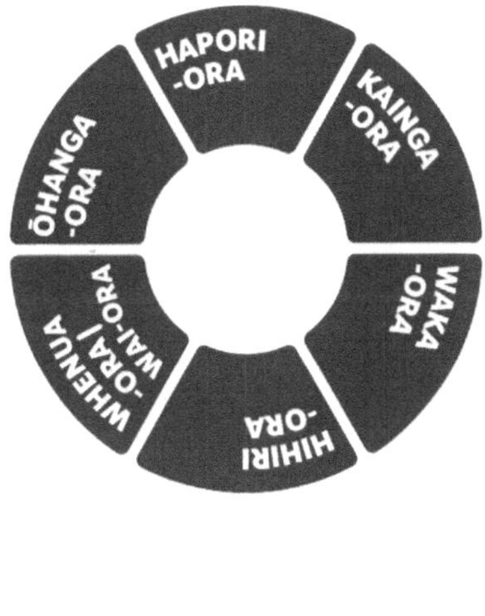

Fig. 7.2 Simplified mauri ora assessment tool. From Dombroski et al. (2022, p. 14)

in common, communities can also emerge from being together in a shared place (or commons) that individuals collectively come to care for (J.K. Gibson-Graham 2006; Larsen and Johnson 2017). The majority of LiVS-supported projects in this research have outcomes in hapori ora (connected communities). The majority of the arts-based projects were in this category too.

Ōhanga ora—Circular Bioeconomies. I categorised the organisation/ project as returning ōhanga ora if it contributed to sustainable economic wellbeing. Usually, this was because it enabled people to make a livelihood, or contributed to some form of circular economy (redesign, reuse, and recycling of materials) (Kirchherr et al. 2017). For example, Rekindle teaches people how to reuse, repair and repurpose discarded objects or make them into crafted objects of purpose and art, and GapFiller's Dance-o-Mat was a repurposed washing machine. Many of the LiVS-supported projects in this research have outcomes in ōhanga ora (circular bioeconomies).

Whenua ora | wai ora—Regenerative Ecosystems. I categorised the organisation/project returning whenua & wai ora if it contributed to environmental wellbeing. Environmental wellbeing is not just about minimising damage to the environment, but about contribution to

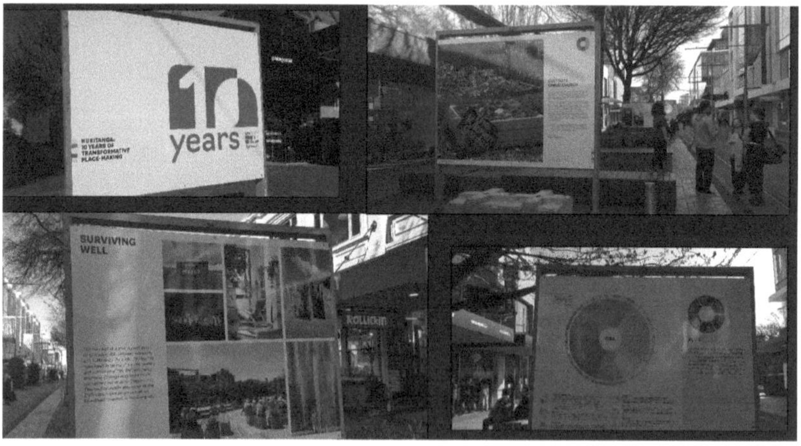

Fig. 7.3 Exhibition montage

regeneration (Reed 2007). For example, Cultivate Christchurch actively regenerated the ecosystem of their LiVS site in Peterborough Street, building up some 30 centimetres of soil, while Aoake's performance *Meat Prize* challenged consumption practices and the environmental damage of meat consumption. Some of the LiVS-supported projects in this research have outcomes in whenua and wai ora.

Waka ora—Active Accessible Transport. I categorised the organisation/project returning 'waka ora' if it contributed to active and accessible transport in the city or used active or accessible transport as part of the project itself. Active and accessible transport includes public transport systems, as well as the infrastructure that supports active modes of transport such as, footpaths, cycleways, bus shelters, and bike stands (Keall et al. 2018). For example, Big Street Bikers, place their 'Locky Dock' bike stands in LiVS locations around the city, allowing secure, free bike parking funded partly via the advertising on their stands. The outcome here is improved access to active transport. Cultivate uses electric bikes to pick up green waste bins and make vegetable deliveries. A small number of LiVS-supported projects in this research had outcomes in 'waka ora', usually alongside other outcomes.

Hihiri ora—Ecological Energy. I categorised the organisation/project returning 'hihiri ora' if it contributed to more widespread use of alternative low-carbon energy systems, or reduced fossil fuel usage. For example, Jess from Mamacita's considered the different types of cooking energy and tried to balance the use of fossil fuels with renewable energies. Very few LiVS-supported projects in this research had outcomes in hihiri ora.

Kainga ora—Living Carbon Storing Buildings. I categorised the organisation/project returning kainga ora if it contributed to, resulted in, or used more renewable building design in the city, or encouraged culturally relevant design and landscapes (including beautification and public art). For example, The Green Lab's plant-filled temporary coworking spaces and Watch This Space which resulted in striking murals across the city. Many of the LiVS-supported projects in this research have outcomes in kainga ora, contributing to place-making of Ōtautahi Christchurch following the earthquakes.

The assessment matrix was a simple Word document, that was later developed into a visual published in our report (Dombroski et al. 2023). One of the limitations is that neither the CEROI nor the Mauri

Ora Compass were necessarily only about investments/intentions and returns/outcomes, and the Mauri Ora Compass was not designed as an assessment tool but as a planning tool. However, in the scope of the exhibition and the short book we were producing, it served as a visual prompt to help us 'see' the holistic nature of an assessment through the different kinds of wellbeing it invited us to consider.

Presenting the Evaluation

The assessment was first developed into an exhibition and booklet, celebrating 10 years of LiVS' work (Dombroski et al. 2022). This exhibition was held on Ōtautahi Christchurch's Cashel Street (Fig.7.3), which had been the site of temporary LiVS projects including a shopping district made of shipping containers that held the space for many years before the rebuild. The exhibition was not intended to provide a scientific evaluation measuring citizens' wellbeing over ten years, but to evoke a sense of accomplishment, a little nostalgia, and an appreciation for the incredible work so many people had put into the community side of recovery and place-making. As such it featured large, beautiful imagery alongside minimalist text and clear iconography. The kinds of art projects and community interventions that were represented were clearly holistic, as demonstrated by the compass badge with the holistic aspects of mauri ora highlighted against specific projects. We imagined a whole range of city leaders walking past this every day for the 10 days of the exhibition—so much so that we put off the exhibition until more people had returned to office work in the central city and after the winter cold and flu season was finished (September 2022). We wanted people to experience this evaluation in place, and in many ways, with their bodies, rather than just the analytical report-reading mind that might otherwise be invoked.

With the support of colleagues in our wider research programme, we went on to develop a report that laid out the background and evidence for the exhibition and the booklet (Dombroski et al. 2022, 2023). We published the report through our research funder and used a different designer to visually separate this report from the more celebratory booklet and exhibition. The visual effect we were going for in this output was one of formal academic evaluation and validation of the partnership approach we had taken—common in community-led development circles, but less common in consultancy-driven evaluations. For me, this was the final point in the decade of work leading up to this moment—but in many ways, I felt dissatisfied with not being able to really develop something robust and reusable. But perhaps, as I reflect below, this is indeed the point.

Lessons Learned: Wellbeing Assessments and the Participatory Arts

In many ways, this experiment with evaluation was felt by all of us to be merely communicating what those of us who had engaged with the work of LiVS already knew: it was clearly wellbeing enhancing. But what the experiment was about was community organisations having some control of the evaluation process, to answer the questions posed by Irene at the beginning of this chapter but in a way that brought the organisation and its community along for the process. Her question was: how to measure and communicate the value of what LiVS does—and the art interventions it supports—so that it can be heard by others? The starting point of this question assumes there is value in the work by virtue of the fact that people continue to find meaning in investing huge amounts of time and energy into both the brokering work (of LiVS) and the initiatives themselves. This is a starting point I share.

What then is to be said of the final evaluation of LiVS? The role of the arts in supporting wellbeing, particularly in the context of post-earthquake recovery, is certainly evident in the work of LiVS. By providing spaces for creative expression and community engagement, LiVS has enabled a diverse range of projects that contribute to the holistic wellbeing of Ōtautahi Christchurch, particularly in the areas of connecting community, regenerating landscapes, and wellbeing-enhancing buildings.

And what is my evaluation of this work developing methods for evaluation? The use of qualitative assessment tools such as CEROI and the Mauri Ora Compass has been instrumental in documenting these impacts, experimenting with a holistic assessment of the value generated by arts initiatives. But it still leaves much to be desired. I see a disconnect between using the two frameworks of CEROI and Mauri Ora, which I have really used to my own ends in ways the authors have not intended. In many ways, the CEROI is about 'hacking' the return on investment narrative with the kinds of monetary calculations performed by Petrescu et al. (2021), and the Mauri Ora Compass is better suited to planning and directing action in the way Yates et al. (2022) have used it. Yet in many ways, this reflects the ongoing problem of trying to evaluate and measure holistic wellbeing outcomes of any art or community intervention. In some ways, it is better to 'muck in' (Wright 2017), to just begin and get on with it, even as it is imperfect and frustrating.

What I can hold on to is this: The work began from the starting point of partnership, and sustained academic attention to the kinds of research questions being asked by communities, including artists and creatives. For myself, the commitment is to create methods, outputs, and interventions that enable communities, funders, and decision-makers to recognise and invest in the arts as a vital component of holistic wellbeing and resilience. The arts allow us to access parts of ourselves that are holistic and more-than-rational, to tap into what it means to live a good life, be an Earth being, and to be moved and connected with others and ourselves. Creating methods that allow us to see and acknowledge those contributions is vital in an economic landscape where rationalist individualism is embedded into decision-making structures. This holistic valuing and translation work is the work I will continue to do as I move forward in community-led action research.

Acknowledgements I acknowledge the many contributions of my colleagues and community partners over the last decade into this work. There was too many to name individually, but you will find them in the acknowledgements or author lists for projects referenced. Funding for the different projects mentioned has been provided by Ministry of Business, Innovation, and Enterprise, The Royal Society Te Aparangi, and the George Sevicke Jones Trust.

References

Clare, Grace, Gradon Diprose, Louise Lee, Phil Bremer, Sheila Skeaff, and Miranda Mirosa. 2023. Measuring the impact of food rescue: A social return on investment analysis. *Food Policy* 117: 102454

Cloke, Paul, and David Conradson. 2018. Transitional organisations, affective atmospheres and new forms of being-in-common: Post-disaster recovery in Christchurch, New Zealand. *Transactions of the Institute of British Geographers* 43 (3): 360–376. https://doi.org/10.1111/tran.12240

Cloke, Paul, David Conradson, Eric Pawson, and Harvey Perkins. 2023. *The Post-Earthquake City: Disaster and Recovery in Christchurch, New Zealand*. New York: Routledge

Dombroski, Kelly, Gradon Diprose, David Conradson, Stephen Healy, and Alison Watkins. 2018. *When Cultivate Thrives: Developing Criteria for Community Economy Return on Investment.* National Science Challenge 11 Building Better Homes, Towns and Cities (Christchurch, NZ). http://www.buildingbetter.nz/publications/contestable_research_projects/Dombroski_et_al_2018_when_cultivate_thrives.pdf. Accessed 23 March 2025

Dombroski, Kelly, Gradon Diprose, David Conradson, Stephen Healy, and Alison F. Watkins. 2019. *Delivering Urban Wellbeing through Transformative Community Enterprise: Final Report.* https://hdl.handle.net/10092/100656. Accessed 23 March 2025

Dombroski, Kelly, Hugh Nicholson, Rachael Shiels, Hannah Watkinson, Amanda Yates, and Life in Vacant Spaces. 2022. *Huritanga: 10 years of transformational place-making.* Christchurch: Life in Vacant Spaces and Building Better Homes Towns and Cities

Dombroski, Kelly, Gradon Diprose, Matthew Scobie, and Amanda Yates. 2023. *Enabling life in vacant spaces: A partnership approach to evaluating holistic wellbeing in disaster recovery contexts.* Building Better Homes, Towns and Cities (Wellington). https://www.communityeconomies.org/publications/reports/enabling-life-vacant-spaces-partnership-approach-evaluating-holistic-wellbeing. Accessed 23 March 2025

Durie, Mason. 1999. Te Pae Māhutonga: a model for Māori health promotion. *Health Promotion Forum of New Zealand Newsletter* 49: 1-8

Gibson-Graham, J. K., Jenny Cameron, and Stephen Healy. 2013. *Take Back the Economy: An ethical guide for transforming our communities.* Minneapolis: University of Minnesota Press

Gibson-Graham, J.K. 2006. *A Postcapitalist Politics.* Minneapolis: University of Minnesota Press

Healy, Stephen, Kelly Dombroski, Gradon Diprose, David Conradson, Joanne McNeill, and Alison Watkins. 2019. More than monitoring: Developing impact measures for transformative social enterprise. Implementing the Sustainable Development Goals: What Role for Social and Solidarity Economy?, UNTFSSE International Conference in Geneva

Kamp, A., C. Brown, T. McMenamin, and V. O'Toole. 2022. *Wellbeing: Global Policies and Perspectives: Insights from Aotearoa New Zealand and Beyond.* Peter Lang

Keall, Michael D., Caroline Shaw, Ralph Chapman, and Philippa Howden-Chapman. 2018. Reductions in carbon dioxide emissions from an intervention to promote cycling and walking: A case study from New Zealand. *Transportation Research Part D: Transport and Environment* 65: 687–696. https://doi.org/10.1016/j.trd.2018.10.004

Kirchherr, Julian, Denise Reike, and Marko Hekkert. 2017. "Conceptualizing the circular economy: An analysis of 114 definitions." *Resources, Conservation and Recycling* 127: 221–232. https://doi.org/10.1016/j.resconrec.2017.09.005

Larsen, Soren C, and Jay T Johnson. 2017. *Being together in place: Indigenous coexistence in a more than human world*. Minneapolis: University of Minnesota Press

Petrescu, Doina, Constantin Petcou, Maliha Safri, and Katherine Gibson. 2021. "Calculating the value of the commons: Generating resilient urban futures." *Environmental Policy and Governance* 31 (3): 159–174

Reed, Bill. 2007. Shifting from 'sustainability' to regeneration. *Building Research & Information* 35 (6): 674–680. https://doi.org/10.1080/09613210701475753

Wright, Sarah. 2017. Critique as delight, theory as praxis, mucking in. *Geographical Research* 55 (3): 338–343. https://doi.org/10.1111/1745-5871.12207

Yates, Amanda Monehu. 2021. Transforming geographies: Performing Indigenous-Māori ontologies and ethics of more-than-human care in an era of ecological emergency. *New Zealand Geographer* 77 (2): 101–113. https://doi.org/10.1111/nzg.12302

Yates, Amanda Monehu. 2022. Hurihanga mo te mauri ora: Braided rivers and pluriversal planetary wellbeing. In *Wellbeing: global policies and perspectives*, ed. A. Kamp, C. Brown, T. McMenamin and V. O'Toole, 243–265. Peter Lang

Yates, Amanda Monehu, Kelly Dombroski, and Rita Dionisio. 2023. Dialogues for wellbeing in an ecological emergency: Wellbeing-led governance frameworks and transformative Indigenous tools. *Dialogues in Human Geography* 13 (2): 268–287. https://doi.org/10.1177/20438206221102957

Yates, Amanda Monehu, Maibritt Pedersen Zari, Sibyl Bloomfield, Andrew Burgess, Charles Walker, Kathy Waghorn, Priscila Besen, Nick Sargent, and Fleur Palmer. 2022. A transformative architectural pedagogy and tool for a time of converging crises. *Urban Science* 7 (1): 1

CHAPTER 8

Hobson Street Theatre Company: Developing an Evaluation Framework

Rand Hazou, Bronwyn Bent, Joeli Thacker, John Hughes, Richard Nightingale, Leonard Mathews, Kelly Tunui, and Gem McIver

Introduction

The Hobson Street Theatre Company (HSTC) was formed in 2010 when theatre producers Bronwyn Bent and Sally Barnett approached the Auckland City Mission with the idea of hosting weekly drama workshops for those using the services of the Auckland City Mission. The Mission, which has been a feature of Auckland for more than 100 years, provides access to homeless services, food assistance, and health support. Wilf Holt, the Team Leader in Homeless Services at the Mission, supported the initiative

R. Hazou (✉) · J. Thacker · J. Hughes · R. Nightingale · L. Mathews · K. Tunui · G. McIver
Massey University, Albany, New Zealand
e-mail: R.T.Hazou@massey.ac.nz

B. Bent
Auckland, New Zealand
e-mail: bronwyn@flock.nz

M. Mullen et al. (eds.), *Artful Evaluation for Creative Health and Wellbeing*, New Directions in Cultural Policy Research,
https://doi.org/10.1007/978-3-032-17063-7_8

and eventually Borni Te Rongopai Tukiwaho and Amelia Yiakmis joined the creative team to facilitate the weekly theatre drop-in sessions. The HSTC was formed out of community participants attending the theatre drop-in sessions. To date, the sessions have engaged more than 140 participants, with different volunteer and support staff coming and going. Attendance at these sessions has fluctuated over time, but usually there are about 10 participants attending regularly to collaborate on creative work together. The core commitment of the group is to provide an open, relaxed and safe atmosphere where all are welcome. From these drop-in sessions participants have been recruited to work on key theatre projects. Over the last 12 years, the Company has produced around 10 productions and has received several awards (Hazou 2023). These achievements have included travelling to Rotterdam in 2023 to take part in the International Community Arts Festival (ICAF), and, most recently, a production of *Not King Lear* directed by Adrian Jackson for the Auckland Arts Festival in 2023.

Homelessness

A central aspect of the company's vision is to 'use theatre as a way to share the stories of those with experience of living on the street', and to 'foster dialogue on issues that lead to and perpetuate homelessness' (Hazou 2023, 102). The company also aims to demonstrate to audiences that, in the words of one group member, 'Homeless don't mean hopeless' (ibid. 116). In New Zealand, homelessness is defined as 'a living situation where people with no other options to acquire safe and secure housing are: without shelter, in temporary accommodation, sharing accommodation with a household, or living in uninhabitable housing' (Statistics New Zealand 2015). The New Zealand definition recognises 'concealed' homeless living situations which includes people who have no other housing option but to share someone else's accommodation on a temporary basis (Edgar and Meert 2006). This might include 'couch surfing' or sleeping with extended whānau (family) in overcrowded rooms. Homelessness is not just the absence of shelter, it is 'the absence of safe, secure and habitable shelter' (Rua et al. 2019, 10).

In 2021, it was estimated that there were 102,123 people who were severely housing deprived, which was nearly 2.2% of the population (Amore et al. 2021, 4). More recently, a report from the OECD suggests

New Zealand has one of the highest rates of homelessness in the developed world depending on which definition of homelessness is used. New Zealand is rated seventh among the 38 member countries for the number of people per 10,000 who are homeless, as defined by either sleeping rough or in emergency accommodation (Coughlan 2024). The global pandemic and an economic recession have worsened the situation, leading the Wellington City Missioner Murray Edridge to report that New Zealand's homelessness problem has reached a scale not seen since the Depression and the World Wars (Wells 2024). Moreover, it is important to note how the issue of homelessness impacts New Zealand's Indigenous population. According to a survey on regional homelessness conducted in September 2018, 43% of people living without shelter in the Auckland region in Aotearoa, New Zealand, were of Māori ethnicity (Statistica 2024, 223). The overrepresentation of Māori homelessness reflects the ongoing effects of colonisation and discrimination (Groot and Peters 2016). This context helps to highlight the structural inequalities that contribute to and produce homelessness. As Rua et al. (2009, 10) point out, homelessness is not an outcome of individual bad choices or personal failings; it is the result of whānau (families) living under-resourced lives, and as such, 'poverty and homelessness are intrinsically connected'. Understanding this context helps to frame the approach to HSTC's practice and evaluation, as an effort to resist an individualised and problematising approach that situates homeless people themselves as a 'problem' that must be addressed. This context has informed HSTC's efforts to develop practice and evaluation that shift the focus from deficit models predicated on problematising individual behaviour, to strength-based approaches informed by holistic and communal understandings.

Design Workshops and Theory of Change

A key feature of HSTC's work is its engagement with the 'street' and with the community accessing services from the Auckland City Mission. As such, they are often facilitating theatre workshops and projects with a community impacted by multiple forms of precarity.

Despite cast members being paid,[1] participants often struggle with health issues impacting their ability to memorise lines. They might also be contending with diminished concentration from a lack of adequate food or sleep. Within this context, just 'showing up' can be an important marker of success. However, the HSTC aims to encourage individual self-expression and community cohesion through creative participation. While the company does not explicitly support people to find housing, employment, or connect with family and friends, underscoring the work of the company is a focus on increasing the self-confidence and wellbeing of participants through creative engagement as a necessary condition for navigating other aspects of their lives. How participants engage with HSTC is rarely a linear process, and different individuals make progress overcoming various challenges impacting their lives at different rates. These considerations impact on the company and its ability to evaluate aspects of its work as well as how 'data' is collected. Because of these factors, a theory of change model was suggested by Bronwyn Bent as the most appropriate one to evaluate programmes.

A theory of change is a 'description of a social change initiative that shows how early changes relate to more intermediate changes and then to longer-term change' (Ellis et al. 2011, 2). In relation to applied theatre, Cahill (2018, 180) describes a theory of change as 'a sketch of the anticipated change process' that 'identifies the goals and objectives'. For Cahill, a theory of change 'houses a set of presumptions about what will be done, what is going to work, and what will be accomplished' (ibid.). Importantly, the benefit of a theory of change approach is that it 'puts emphasis on what you want to achieve rather than what you want to do' (Ellis et al. 2011, 4). The decision to incorporate a theory of change into the design of the HSTC evaluation framework was also influenced by the example of Streetwise Opera, a UK organisation that runs music programmes with the homeless community. Streetwise Opera use theory of change in their evaluation practice to provide 'a clear and testable theory about how change occurs', but also to provide a means for evaluating work with 'measurable indicators of success' (Parkinson 2017, 6). Informing the development of Streetwise Opera's evaluation tool was the desire for a

[1] The company has secured arts grant funding for their various public productions over the years which includes budget to pay the company actors. The company has also hired and paid company actors to work as facilitators on various community outreach projects involving weekly workshops and drop-in sessions.

robust system which was 'realistic' given what can be achieved with the resources available to them (ibid.).

In order to develop a theory of change evaluation framework for the HSTC, the company decided to hold two co-design workshops that focused on aspects of wellbeing. This follows Cahill's (2018, 181) suggestion about the need to 'co-construct the theory of change' through a process that involves 'dialogic exchange' about 'progress markers' or the signs or indicators that you might expect to see if a programme or project is on track. The workshops were held at the Auckland City Mission's Homeground—its main facility located in the central city that comprises fully-integrated housing and social services. The first workshop began with company members being asked: *given we have different conceptions of wellbeing, what does wellbeing mean to you?* This resulted in different suggestions, including things like 'mental health', 'physical and mental strength', 'having energy', and 'just showing up', among others. The focus here was on identifying criteria of success that the group values which are connected to conceptions of wellbeing that the company could include in framework to help them evaluate their work. Following a theory of change approach (Ellis et al. 2011), company members were asked to think about how they might identify each criterion in a rehearsal or workshop session and what this might look like in the short term, medium, and long term. These were used to create a draft model that was taken back to company members for further development at a second workshop three weeks later.

The second workshop introduced the model of Indigenous health Te Whare Tapa Whā or the House of Four Sides (Durie 1994), as a useful model onto which the various indicators of success mentioned by the company could be mapped. Both sessions were facilitated by Rand Hazou who had previously worked with the company on creative and teaching projects. There were six company members present at both sessions. Importantly, four of the company members attending the workshops identify as Māori. This, as well as the fact that issues of homelessness disproportionately impact Māori and as a result, the precarious community that HSTC engages with, informed the discussions of the workshops and the design of HSTC's evaluation model, which will be explored in more detail in the following sections.

Engaging with Conceptions of Wellbeing and Hauora

The first workshop provoked participants to think about criteria for evaluating their work that were linked to aspects of wellbeing. Members of the company were initially invited to think about potential differences between conceptions of wellbeing and the Māori notion of hauora. Within the health sector in Aotearoa, hauora has been defined as 'a Māori perspective of health and wellbeing', and the use of this term has created a space for a Māori voice within Māori health policy (Heaton 2011, 101). Hauora can be traced to the pūrakau (narratives) that underpin the Māori worldview. It is described as the supernatural hau (breath) of ora (life) given to the first female Hine-ahu-one, the progenitor of humanity, who was shaped from the earth by Tāne-mahuta, the Māori god of the forests and birds (Heaton 2016, 461–462). Given that, within the Māori world, Hine-ahu-one is considered the progenitor of humanity, Heaton suggests that hauora can be described as 'the animation of life' (ibid, 462). Reweti and colleagues (2023) provide a useful explanation of the individual terms that comprise the word in order to explain its full meaning:

> One of the meanings of hau is the vital essence embodied in all persons and living things according to a Māori worldview. An expression of hau in people is breath. Ora means to be alive, to be well. The word hauora can therefore be defined as the totality of vital elements that contribute to a flourishing, dynamic and vital spirit of life. (13)

Hauora offers a holistic understanding of a person's health that includes aspects of spirituality, cultural identity, and connection to whānau (extended family or social grouping) and the natural world (ibid.). For the first HSTC design workshop, the aim of prompting company members to consider notions of hauora was to ensure that an evaluation model that we developed was not limited by Western notions of wellbeing. While most of the members present at the design workshop were Māori, the discussion was facilitated by Rand Hazou, a non-Māori scholar and theatre-maker. As such, the facilitation was conducted while being mindful of the dangers of misappropriating Indigenous understandings or reinforcing literal translations of Māori concepts. Elsewhere, Heaton points out the dangers of literal translations of Māori words and concepts and their co-option by dominant culture. As Heaton has noted, 'translating hauora simplistically as health and physical wellbeing potentially debases metaphorical and etymological ways of knowing' (Heaton 2011, 104). Rather than providing simplistic or reductive responses to notions of hauora in the first workshop, HSTC members' initial conceptions of wellbeing seemed to emphasise the social interconnections that are engendered through the group's engagement with participatory arts. When asked for criteria of success linked to aspects of wellbeing, members of the company initially suggested things like 'movement', 'strength of community', and that 'people feel connected and that they can rely on each other'. Already a nuance was emerging in the discussion that seemed to shift the focus from individual notions of health to more communal or social conceptions of wellbeing.

A few of the initial conceptions of wellbeing that were offered in the first workshop are worth noting here to demonstrate the nuance with which aspects of wellbeing were being conceived and related specifically the street community that the company engages with. For example, in the initial discussion, members identified 'confidence' as a key element of emotional wellbeing. Prompted for more detail, Gemma suggested this was about being 'confident to be vulnerable' which she later elaborated as feeling 'psychologically safe'. Underpinning this discussion of confidence as a marker of emotional or psychological wellbeing was an understanding that it can also translate as a community participant sitting confidently but quietly in a workshop or at least not feeling any pressure to necessarily 'perform'. In another example, long-time member of the company Richard mentioned the importance of 'stepping out of oneself as a character' and the importance of 'characterisation'. When prompted for further detail, Richard explained that this was about 'stepping outside of the ego'. This was understood as the opportunity that performance offers to move 'beyond the self', which Richard later described as 'unselfing' by referencing the work of philosopher Iris Murdoch (2023).

A discussion of 'humour' as an indicator of wellbeing provoked mixed responses. At first, members suggested that humour can be a 'mask' that can be used as a barrier to avoid vulnerability and as a barrier that might inhibit the establishment of genuine connections required for creative collaboration. However, company members also suggested that humour and the ability of members to 'rib each other' and laugh at each other was often an indication of levels of safety in the workshop or rehearsal room.

Another aspect of the discussion was the notion of developing connections between participants. Bronwyn recalled a member who joined the drop-in sessions who literally could not make eye contact and would sit in the sessions with his eyes closed. Eventually, this participant got to a point where they felt comfortable enough to make eye contact with others. The group agreed that this simple physiological shift could constitute an important indicator of wellbeing and success for the workshops or projects involving participants from precarious backgrounds. Joeli expanded a bit on the notion of 'showing up' as a key indicator of wellbeing for the group. He suggested that, for the City Mission whānau (family) or people from a marginalised or trauma-based community, it can be really intimidating for people to let go and be able to play. This aspect is particularly relevant to HSTC's constituent community who are often struggling with housing, health, and sobriety issues. For this precarious community, 'showing up' becomes a key marker of success for the company. Moreover, given the company's connection to the Auckland City Mission, the group also mentioned the provision of basic material needs for participants in the form of food and tea and coffee at workshops and drop-in sessions. Caring for the basic physical needs of participants was considered an essential aspect of the company's approach and a worthwhile criterion to evaluate its workshops or programmes.

Engaging with Te Whare Tapa Whā: The House of Four Sides

When drafting up the company's initial ideas and feedback, most of the qualities identified by the company in the first design workshop fit into the broad areas of 'mental', 'physical', and 'social' categories of wellbeing. At the second workshop, the company were invited to think about a fourth aspect of wellbeing in relation to spirit or wairua. This was informed by a model of Māori health developed by Sir Mason Durie (1994) called Te Whare Tapa Whā (The House of Four Sides). This Indigenous model of wellbeing uses the metaphor of the wharenui or meeting house with four walls or sides (Fig. 8.1). These walls include taha tinana (physical health), taha wairua (spiritual health), taha hinengaro (mental health), and taha whānau (social health). Within this holistic model, each wall is integral to the integrity of the entire building. The model was familiar to the participants as it has become popular as a tool for thinking about

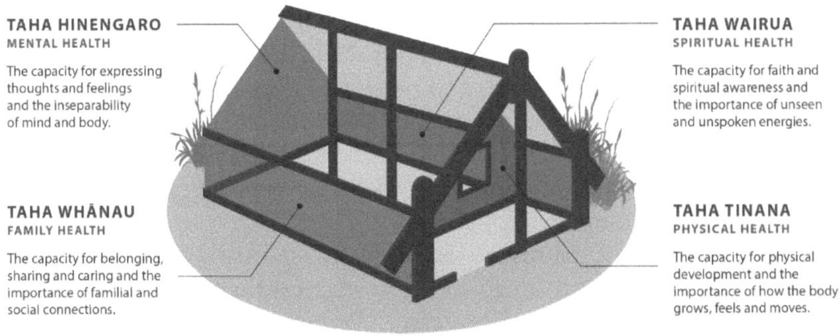
TAHA HINENGARO
MENTAL HEALTH
The capacity for expressing thoughts and feelings and the inseparability of mind and body.
TAHA WAIRUA
SPIRITUAL HEALTH
The capacity for faith and spiritual awareness and the importance of unseen and unspoken energies.
TAHA WHĀNAU
FAMILY HEALTH
The capacity for belonging, sharing and caring and the importance of familial and social connections.
TAHA TINANA
PHYSICAL HEALTH
The capacity for physical development and the importance of how the body grows, feels and moves.

Fig. 8.1 Te Whare Tapa Whā or The House of Four Sides—a holistic model of Māori Health developed by Sir Mason Durie based on the metaphor of the wharenui or meeting house. Image credit: Jeanne Leclercq (2021)

a holistic approach in the provision of health, counselling, and sobriety programmes offered by organisations such as City Mission.

In the second design workshop, participants were asked to think about aspects of 'wairua' or spiritual health which might include some qualities such as 'Un-Selfing', the 'ability to remove personal masks', 'moving beyond oneself', and 'creating perspective'. These were all qualities that the company offered in the first workshop session, but which were discussed mainly in relation to mental health. After introducing the model of Te Whare Tapa Whā for the company a discussion of 'shift in perspective' was explained as an individual moving beyond a focus on their own individuality in the short term, to being more proactive in helping to establish connections in the long term. In some ways the discussion of this aspect of spiritual health ultimately crosses over into aspects of taha whānau and its focus on social connections which is indicative of the holistic approach to wellbeing in which the different sides of a person's wellbeing are interconnected and inform each other.

Following this discussion, we attempted to map the qualities emerging in the first workshop onto the Te Whare Tapa Whā model (Table 8.1). Most of the criteria or values fit relatively easily. Some qualities shifted to a different taha (wall) or aspect to line up with the model. The company discussed certain qualities that might be included in the more expansive notion of different sides or taha of wellbeing. For example, as an aspect of Taha hinengaro—mental wellbeing—the group discussed the development of communication and listening skills. This was prompted when thinking about how confidence and personal development over time can lead to a participant speaking calmly and without anger in workshops or drop-ins. The discussion also considered whether there were other qualities of wairua or spiritual health, such as compassion, that might be articulated as part of an evaluation model.

The final aspect of the discussion involved aspects of creative integrity and the company's desire to focus on artistic excellence and the professional development of the performers. Embedded within Durie's original model was the foundational notion of the whenua or land on which the wharenui or meeting house sits (Higgins and Goodall 2021, 3). For the HSTC participants, the artistic and creative integrity of the company was discussed in terms of the papa or floor of the whare. This was an important addition to the company's considerations of how they would evaluate their work. Ultimately, the various criteria for success rested on the creative ambitions of the company to provide moments of creative inspiration, opportunities for actor development, and aspirations to push creative boundaries and innovate theatrical forms in production. Moreover, while the company has always insisted on paying members for theatre projects, a longer-term appraisal of their work also aspired to ensure that members could be employable and that those who aspire to be paid professional actors could and should be supported in achieving this goal. This aspect of creative integrity was added to the evaluation framework as the floor on which the whare or house sits.

How HSTC Might Apply the Evaluation Framework

The HSTC have several ethical and practical considerations for how their evaluation framework might be applied and what the process of 'data collection' might entail. The company is conscious that many of their community participants have had the experience of institutions requiring data from them and then not always knowing what happens to that data. HSTC is also aware that there may be distrust and suspicion about Pākehā-led research and evaluation. The term 'research' is inextricably linked to European imperialism and colonialism, and as Māori scholar Linda Tuhiwai Smith has noted, the term 'research' is 'probably one of the dirtiest words in the indigenous world's vocabulary' (Smith 2012, 54). The HSTC want participants to feel empowered and that they have

Table 8.1 The Hobson Street Theatre company evaluation framework

Quality	*Short Term*	*Medium Term*	*Long Term*
Taha hinengaro: Mental Health			
Cultivating Presence and Engagement	Showing Up—Just being in the room	Actively Participating	Leading Sessions
Enhancing Play and Joy	Laughter Shift in Mood	Sharing & being vulnerable Spontaneity	Developing confidence Personal growth Accepting that it is ok to experience troughs or dips
Developing communication and listening	Relaxed bodies Making eye contact Contributing vocally and physically	Active listening Vocal projection. Speaking clearly and calmly	Giving space to others Sense of whānau connection Aligning with the kaupapa of the company
Taha tinana: Physical Health			
Showing up and Motivation	Showing up	Actively participating in setting up sessions	Organising and motivating others
Energy and Strength	Basic physical needs are met No hunger or thirst	Developing energy and stamina	Actively managing health to support performance
Movement and Flexibility	Having a go. Participating in physical warmups	Leading a warmup or exercise	Supporting and being aware of others' physical limitations and abilities
Taha whanau: Family Health			
Enhancing Inclusion and Non-judgement	Welcoming others No sexist, racist, ableist language	Understanding and working with people's strengths	Taking care of audiences

(continued)

Table 8.1 (continued)

Quality	*Short Term*	*Medium Term*	*Long Term*
Cultivating Trust	Not forcing anyone to do anything they don't want to	Cultivating willingness Maintaining connections and trust with wider company members	Trust as integral in recruiting other participants
Taha wairua: Spiritual Health			
Creating Perspective	Shifting from focus on 'me' to focus on 'others'	Aware of one's own energy and affect on others	Being intentional in establishing connections
Enhancing Compassion and Communion	Being open and accepting of others	Having compassion for oneself	Aware of one's own responsibility to create community connections and communion
Papa/Ground: Creative Integrity			
Artistic excellence and Performer Development	Moments of Creative Spark and Inspiration	Active aspirations for improvement Developing Voice, Physicality, and Acting Skills	It's a Job! Meaningful employment Pushing boundaries in terms of form and content Finding innovative forms that reflects the collective

control over their data and know what is happening with it. The company are committed to ensuring that all participants are able to rescind their information at any time and that all reports and other evaluation materials will anonymise/de-identify participants unless they would prefer not to be.

In terms of 'data collection', the HSTC are also conscious that some participants have different levels of comfort with writing, so it is critical that responses can be provided in different ways enabling everyone to participate. It may also be off-putting for new participants, especially at casual, drop-in sessions, to be presented with a form to fill out, so a mix of different evaluation tools, some suggestions of which are listed below, which do not always require people to fill out forms is useful. Furthermore, a variety of information-gathering methods means that the data can have a richness and depth that one method may not supply. For these reasons, the company has suggested the following data collection methods where the evaluation framework can guide contributions and discussions.

Sharing a pou: The company has developed a culturally informed protocol for opening and closing sessions which was introduced by founding company member Borni Te Rongopai Tukiwaho and involves each participant setting a 'pou'. This was introduced to the company. In the Māori world this often translates as 'post' or 'upright support' and can be found as carved central posts upholding traditional meeting houses or wharenui. At the start of each HSTC session, all participants are asked to share in two words or fewer what emotion or thought they are brining into the room. This could be 'excitement', 'sadness', 'tiredness', 'anticipation', or even current preoccupations such as 'thinking of my sister', or 'my pain in my shoulder'. This process is repeated at the end of each session with everyone saying how they currently feel or whether the thought they shared at the start of the session has shifted or changed. The distance between these two pou can be a useful gauge of how a session has gone. The development of HSTC's evaluation framework offers the company a means to bring further nuance to these pou by asking participants to share something that connects with one of the four taha or aspects of wellbeing.

Focus Groups: Another method the HSTC might employ are the use of focus groups involving longer discussion session to discuss what is working and what might need to be improved with each programme or project. Again, the HSTC evaluation framework might be used to inform discussions by offering participants goals that the company are aiming to achieve. The intention is to have facilitators record the notes so that they can feed into the company's reports and reporting mechanisms.

Continuum Exercise: One method that might be used to elicit both verbal and non-verbal feedback from participants is to use a continuum exercise that allows participants to place themselves on an imaginary scale in a room where one side of the room designates 'strongly agree' and the other 'strongly disagree'. Participants can be asked to place themselves on the imaginary scale in response to the key criteria related to the different taha or aspects of wellbeing informing the HSTC's evaluation model (Table 8.2). For example, for, a facilitator might ask participants to arrange themselves in the room from 'strongly agree' to 'strongly disagree' in response to 'feeling playful', or 'feeling included', or 'feeling inspired'. This approach allows the participants and the facilitator to get a clear visual representation of how participants are feeling in the room in response to key criteria. This can be a potentially useful method to elicit feedback on a workshop or a project.

The continuum exercise and focus group could be useful tools to build up a picture of how the HSTC is progressing over a number of years, in order to be able to track how things have changed over time. An annual review of HSTC would be a useful way to compile all the various forms of monitoring and be able to compare it year-on-year. This report might predominately be used by company members to reflect upon programmes with a view to making improvements in their delivery. A secondary purpose might also involve using this feedback to report back to funders, partner organisations, and supporters.

Table 8.2 Prompts that can be used in a continuum exercise where participants are asked to place themselves on an imaginary scale and where one side of the room designates 'strongly agree' and the opposing side 'strongly disagree'

Taha hinengaro: Mental Health	· feeling playful · feeling joy · communicating well
Taha tinana: Physical Health	· Feeling motivated · Feeling physically healthy and strong
Taha whānau: Family Health	· Feeling included · Feeling safe
Taha wairua: Spiritual Health	· Feeling present and aware · Feeling compassion
Papa/Ground: Creative Integrity	· Feeling inspired · Feeling you have developed creative skills (Acting, Singing, Writing)

Conclusion

When members of the Hobson Street Theatre Company were asked to reflect on the title of this book, the notion of the 'artful' initially conjured up negative connotations. One member who previously worked as a bookkeeper commented that if the term 'artful' was applied in financial accounting it would suggest someone was 'cooking the books'—hiding or manipulating the financial health of a company or business. Another member suggested the word conjured up suggestions of deceiving or manipulating an audience through artistic practice. This led to an acknowledgement that acting itself has a long history of being associated with lying or pretending but that HSTC's intention with performance is not to deceive but rather to use the artifice and the craft of theatre to encourage audiences to suspend their disbelief, and to challenge audience preconceptions, in order to move the audience emotionally and experientially.

With this acknowledgement, the discussion quickly turned to a conversation about Jack Dawkins, better known as 'the Artful Dodger', a character in Charles Dickens's 1838 novel *Oliver Twist*. The Artful Dodger is a nickname that refers to the character's skill as a pickpocket and the term has become an idiom describing a person who engages in skilful deception. It is perhaps unsurprising that a company that aims to challenge misconceptions about the street community would think of a street urchin when prompted to engage with the notion of the artful. One member of the company commented at length on the character of the Artful Dodger, noting that he is a character that survives the street by using his wits and his wiles. This led to an acknowledgement by HSTC members that there is a common misconception that a lot of the members of the street community are criminals or people that engage in criminal activity. Indeed, a central aim of the HSTC is to use theatre to challenge these kinds of negative stereotypes about the street community. Ultimately, the HSTC's discussion framed 'artful evaluation' as a method for the company to evaluate its own work that privileges notions of careful construction and skilful artifice that connects with the aims of the company to care for the wellbeing of its members and the wider community.

Constructing the evaluation model and writing this chapter have, in some ways, constituted an artful sleight of hand. The process has empowered the company to shift the focus of evaluation and for the group to set out what they consider to be valuable in their artistic endeavours rather than adhering to the values and agendas of external funding bodies or government agencies. A simple but poignant example in the evaluation model that the company have developed is how laughter is a measure of success in a production, something that is important to the company but a feature that wouldn't necessarily be an outcome prioritised by an external agency or body.

In writing this chapter, HSTC's efforts to develop practice and evaluation constitute an artful sleight of hand that attempts to shift the focus from deficit models predicated on problematising individual behaviour, to strength-based approaches informed by holistic and communal understandings. The development of this framework provides a method in which HSTC company members have defined their own measures of the 'success' of a project or programme. This self-determination reflects the wider aims of the company to disrupt more typical hierarchical structures. On a practical level, the framework also provides an easily understandable and straightforward way for participants to think about their own progress, and how this contributes to fostering stronger community connections. Ultimately artful evaluation for the HSTC is about how they assess the skilful care they take with their art, with each other, with their wider community.

References

Amore, Kate, Helen Viggers, and Philippa Howden Chapman. 2021. *Severe Housing Deprivation in Aotearoa New Zealand: June 2021 Update*, Wellington: He Kāinga Oranga and the Housing & Health Research Programme, University of Otago.

Cahill, Helen. 2018. Evaluation and the Theory of Change. In *Applied Theatre: Understanding Change*, eds. Kelly Freebody, Michael Balfour, Michael Finneran, and Michael Anderson, 173–186. Cham, Switzerland: Springer.

Coughlan, Thomas. 2024. NZ among world's worst developed countries for homelessness as Chris Bishop says action on Bill English report 'very soon'. *The New Zealand Herald*, 20 May, 2024. https://www.nzherald.co.nz/nz/politics/nz-leads-world-rankings-of-homelessness-as-chris-bishop-says-action-on-bill-english-report-very-soon/5IJECITTM5BH3AEYQXQ5CPV2F4/

Durie, Mason. 1994. *Whaiora: Māori Health Development*. Auckland: Oxford University Press

Edgar, Bill, and Henk Meert. 2006. Fifth review of statistics on homelessness in Europe. Brussels: European Federation of National Organisations Working

with the Homeless. https://www.feantsaresearch.org/download/5-2006449618011929240409.pdf. Accesssed 25 March 2025.
Ellis, Jean, Diana Parkinson, and Avan Wadia. 2011. Making Connections: Using a theory of change to develop planning and evaluation. Charities Evaluation Services. Accessed 7 April 2025: https://www.oneeastmidlands.org.uk/sites/default/files/library/index.pdf
Groot, Shiloh and Evelyn J. Peters. 2016. Indigenous Homelessness: New Zealand Context. In *Indigenous Homelessness: Perspectives from Canada, Australia, and New Zealand*, eds.Evelyn Peters and Julia Christensen, 323–330. Canada: University of Manitoba Press.
Hazou, Rand. 2023. Performing precarity and transilience: The Hobson Street Theatre Company. *Australasian Drama Studies* 83: 102–130.
Heaton, Sharyn. 2011. The co-opting of 'hauora' into curricula. Cur*riculum Matters* 7: 99–117. https://search.informit.org/doi/abs/10.3316/informit.709725170648724
Heaton, Sharyn. 2016. The Juxtaposition of Māori Words with English Concepts. 'Hauora, Well-Being' as Philosophy. *Educational Philosophy and Theory* 50 (5): 460–68. https://doi.org/10.1080/00131857.2016.1167583
Higgins, Joanna, and Suskya Goodall. 2021. Transforming the Wellbeing Focus in Education: A Document Analysis of Policy in Aotearoa New Zealand. *International Journal of Qualitative Studies on Health and Well-being* 16 (1): 1–14. https://doi.org/10.1080/17482631.2021.1879370
Murdoch, Iris. 2023. *The Sovereignty of Good*. United Kingdom: Taylor & Francis
Parkinson, Diana. 2017. Evaluating arts projects with people who have experienced homelessness: Streetwise Opera's approach. Streetwise Opera and With One Voice. https://artshomelessint.com/wp-content/uploads/2021/04/2017-12-_-Arts-Homelessness-Evaluation-Guide-by-Streetwise-Opera-commissioned-by-WOV.pdf. Accessed 25 March 2025.
Reweti, Angelique, Felicity Ware, and Hoani Moriarty. 2023. A tangata whenua (people of the land) approach to conceptualising Māori health and wellbeing. *Global Health Promotion* 30 (2): 11–18. https://doi.org/10.1177/17579759221113094
Rua, Mohi, Darrin Hodgetts, Ottilie Emma Elisabeth Stolte, Delta King, William Cochrane, Thomas Stubbs, Rolinda Karapu et al. 2019. Precariat Māori households today: The need to reorient policy to cultivate more humane understandings of whānau in need. *Ngā Pae o Te Māramatanga Te Arotahi Series* 2: 1–16. https://researchcommons.waikato.ac.nz/server/api/core/bitstreams/1ebfa9f4-4cf3-4dde-bcf7-d2dff91a4e11/content
Smith, Linda Tuhiwai. 2012. *Decolonizing Methodologies: Research and Indigenous Peoples*. Bloomsbury Academic & Professional.

Statistics New Zealand, 2015. New Zealand Definition of Homelessness: Update. *Statistics New Zealand/Tatauranga Aotearoa*. https://www.stats.govt.nz/assets/Uploads/Retirement-of-archive-website-project-files/Methods/New-Zealand-definition-of-homelessness/nz-definition-homelessness-2015-update.pdf. Accessed 25 March 2025.

Statistica. 2024. Distribution of homeless population in Auckland New Zealand 2018 by ethnicity. *Statista Research Department*. https://www.statista.com/statistics/1028989/new-zealand-homeless-population-in-auckland-by-ethnicity/. Accessed 25 March 2025.

Wells, Imogen. 2024. NZ's homelessness worst 'in living memory'. Stuff. 17 July 2024. https://www.stuff.co.nz/nz-news/350342218/nzs-homelessness-worst-living-memory

CHAPTER 9

Project X: Co-Creating a Meaningful Evaluation Framework for a Creative Youth Wellbeing Programme in Aotearoa

Amber Walls and Borni Te Rongopai Tukiwaho

Introduction

In this chapter, we share insights from a participatory research process used to develop a bespoke evaluation framework for Project X. The research was initiated because Project X, a creative programme for young people experiencing mental health challenges, was under pressure from funders to produce evidence of impact using standardised (medical model) evaluation frameworks. The Project X team found these frameworks to be reductionist, deficit-focused, and alienating to participants. The team embarked on research designed to develop a framework that

A. Walls (✉)
Auckland Council, Auckland, New Zealand
e-mail: amber.walls@aucklandcouncil.govt.nz

B. T. R. Tukiwaho
BATS Theatre, Auckland, New Zealand
e-mail: borni@taurimavibes.co.nz

M. Mullen et al. (eds.), *Artful Evaluation for Creative Health and Wellbeing*, New Directions in Cultural Policy Research,
https://doi.org/10.1007/978-3-032-17063-7_9

could articulate 'impacts' in ways that were aligned with participants' aspirations, informed by evidence, credible to funders, and reflective of the unique contribution of arts-based approaches. The research was designed to bring together the project community (young people and partners—arts, health, education, and kaupapa Māori practitioners) to unpack the active ingredients (practices, principles, and change processes) at play in Project X. This process was accompanied by an extensive review of literature and evidence in the wider field of arts, youth, and wellbeing. Ultimately, we produced a Theory of Change (ToC), a principle-based practice framework grounded in the shared perspectives of the project community, and informed by multiple knowledge systems: lived experience, practitioner expertise, Mātauranga Māori (Māori knowledge), theory, research, and evidence.

Our research process was powerful and is worthy of sharing for several reasons. It produced a rich, culturally embedded account of Project X and the conditions which are critical to effective practice. It highlighted some unique contributions of arts participation to youth wellbeing. The process also enabled a deep critique of conceptions of wellbeing, and questions of value, power, and privilege amongst the project community. These insights revealed both the possibilities and limits of Project X and provided a solid foundation to guide the design of a meaningful evaluation framework. Since the challenges encountered by Project X are not unique but are experienced across the arts and wellbeing field (nationally and internationally), our research is highly relevant to other settings. Although our process was facilitated through a collaboration with the University of Auckland and forms part of an in-depth doctoral study,[1] it is highly adaptable and transferable as a more nimble approach across settings. Indeed, members of the research team have used similar processes in other youth initiatives, though the arts-based research methods are distinct to our specific project.

This chapter is written from the perspectives of the lead researcher and the Kaiārahi (guide) to the PhD thesis. Both perspectives are informed

[1] Chapter draws from University of Auckland PhD *Activating The Arts for Youth Wellbeing in Aotearoa: Practices, Principles and Possibilities*. Author Tracy (Amber) Walls (2024). Ethics approval granted from the University of Auckland Human Participants Ethics Committee (UAHPEC) reference number 010758. Supervisors Dr Molly Mullen, Dr Kelsey Deane, Dr Peter O'Connor.

by many years working (separately and occasionally together) as practitioners in the field of participatory arts and community wellbeing. As the lead researcher I (Amber) draw from my visual arts training and a long history working at the intersection between the arts and wellbeing in roles that include artist facilitator, project designer and manager, fundraiser, evaluator, funder, and commissioner. My interest in evaluation is therefore longstanding. However, this research project was born when I was contracted to evaluate the pilot phase of Project X. At the time, I was a recent migrant to Aotearoa (from the UK). I discovered that a persistent challenge I had encountered overseas—a dependence on inappropriate frameworks to 'prove' the value of arts-based approaches to wellbeing—was also prevalent in Aotearoa. I was also acutely aware of the limitations of my Eurocentric lens in the context of this new Pacific landscape. So, I embarked on this research project as a practitioner seeking to find evaluation frameworks that were more attuned to this context.

I (Borni) broker a similar intersection between the arts and wellbeing drawing from my career as a musician/actor/director/producer and my multi-tiered work with arts and wellbeing organisations across Aotearoa. Over the past thirty years I have garnered a plethora of tools and components that have become beneficial in my career from the areas of Community Arts and Wellbeing Brokerage, Wellbeing/Hauora Facilitation and Cultural Competency Consultantancy, and as an Internal Process and Strategic Forecasting Consultant. te ao Māori guidance has a strong influence on how I navigate any project or work I have with any person or organisation. What is often created into these 'guidance frameworks' for organisations are concepts that inherently flow from the teachings of my whakapapa (heritage).

This chapter is organised as follows: First, we describe the challenge of evaluation in relation to Project X. We contextualise and critique this challenge in relation to the wider national and international context. We then describe the participatory research process used in our study and report key insights. We would like to note that Project X specifically seeks to address mental health but throughout this chapter we use the term wellbeing to acknowledge the dependence of mental health on broader wellbeing. We draw from a holistic and socio-ecological conceptualisation of wellbeing aligned with the Pacific perspective that mind, body, spirit, people, place, and planet are interdependent (Anae et al. 2002). Also, we use the term youth as a shorthand for the age range 13–24, whilst acknowledging that this period covers the broad span of adolescence to young adulthood. We acknowledge that not all people within this age span will identify with the term youth, and also that the term itself is highly critiqued and not neutral. We do not have the space to explore these definitions here but feel it important to acknowledge these points.

Project X Context: Youth, Arts, and Mental Health in Aotearoa

When research for Project X began, it was an Auckland-based pilot project offering participatory arts for young people aged 13–24. All participants were experiencing mental distress, including diagnosed experiences of depression, anxiety, psychosis, and/or addiction. Most were introduced to the project via specialist mental health or addiction services with occasional self-referral. In Aotearoa there is over-representation of Māori, Pacific, migrant, and rainbow young people in the mental health system (Government Inquiry into Mental Health and Addictions 2018), and this was reflected in the demographics of the project cohort.

Project X offered a year-round programme of weekly multi-artform participatory workshops, with four terms each year. Each term functioned as a distinct series, attended by around eight young people with continuation over more than one term welcomed. Different projects targeted groups with more closely aligned age ranges (such as 13–15, 15–17, or 18–24). Each term was facilitated by the Project X Coordinator and creative practitioners drawn from a team of freelancers whose expertise spanned visual arts, digital and literary arts, music, and dance. Activities included practical artmaking (both individual and group projects), interspersed with group critical reflection (discussion), social elements such as shared kai (food), and inclusive practices such as Tikanga (Māori cultural practices), and use of pronouns to acknowledge rainbow identities. Activities took place in a variety of community locations but primarily two arts studios. Despite providing a referral service utilised by public health, social, and education providers, Project X was reliant on a short-term grant from philanthropic sources. Continuation beyond the pilot phase was perceived as dependent on proving evidence of positive impact in terms that aligned with health sector investment priorities.

Youth Mental Wellbeing in Aotearoa

Project X was set up to address national concerns about youth mental wellbeing and gaps in practice that had been identified by prior research. Young people in Aotearoa experience high levels of poor mental health (compared with international statistics) which have been on a negative trajectory for over a decade. The 2018 Mental Health and Addictions Inquiry highlighted the profound failure of current approaches for all young people. Challenges were identified as including a lack of access to effective support services, with dominant approaches often described as stigmatising, alienating, culturally unresponsive, and ineffective. This situation is attributed to the historic and persistent dominance of 'big psychiatry': medical model approaches to mental health. Whilst current national strategy highlights more holistic approaches and acknowledges the contribution of a broad range of agencies to health promotion, prevention, and early intervention, investment still privileges clinical treatments such as counselling and medication (Walls 2024).

A reliance on such approaches is problematic for multiple reasons. These approaches emphasise treatment of symptoms in individuals. They fail to address the significant impact of systemic determinants on well-being and are limited in their potential to address complex needs (Freebody et al. 2019). They privilege a psychologised view of poor mental health, which attributes it to individual vulnerability or deficiency. This contributes to the widely documented stigma associated with mental health and further prevents young people from seeking help and accessing support. Psychologised, individually focused approaches draw from a Eurocentric medical model and are misaligned with Pacific conceptualisations of wellbeing (which are holistic and grounded in the interdependence of people and planet as described above). In addition, current approaches are not aligned with young people's perspectives on the complex environmental factors impacting their mental health, including increasingly stressful and risk-laden social contexts, cyberbullying, discrimination, exam pressures, unaffordable housing, insecure employment, and climate change. They are also not consistent with the approaches that young people believe will be most effective in addressing their distress. These include the development of tools for self-awareness and self-care, action on the social determinants, opportunities to be heard and for young people to shape policies and practices, alongside opportunities for socialising, peer support, relaxation, and fun (Fleming et al.

2020). Notably, these perspectives are aligned with best practice twenty-first century approaches identified through international research with young people. In summary, there is an urgent need to re-imagine youth wellbeing and associated responses (Poulton et al. 2020; Walls 2024).

Evaluating the Potential of Youth, Arts, and Mental Wellbeing in Aotearoa

Project X was established to build on the promising potential of arts-based approaches to address these challenges. A rapidly expanding body of international evidence and practice demonstrates that arts participation can be effective in promoting wide-ranging determinants of youth wellbeing across prevention, intervention, and health promotion contexts (Easwaran et al. 2021; Walls 2024). This evidence has supported growth of a diverse, cross-disciplinary, often innovative field of arts practice promoting health and wellbeing. This field is characterised by different (and sometimes conflicted) ways of working, practice histories and paradigms (perspectives). In relation to young people, it builds on traditions as diverse as the youth development field, community arts, critical pedagogy, social justice arts education, social pedagogy, arts therapies (and more). We are unable to unpack this complexity here, but it is important to acknowledge that arts-based approaches to youth wellbeing refer to diverse approaches with different intentions and outcomes.

Evaluation is a hot topic across the arts and wellbeing field. Relevant literature is focused on the need to improve evaluation methods to demonstrate evidence of impact. Despite recent growth, the field remains under-valued, under-resourced, and struggles with lack of credibility. The field is largely populated by small non-government charities (like Project X) whose survival depends on securing income from short-term sources, usually competitive grants from philanthropic, government, and other sources (Critical Research Unit in Applied Theatre 2019). This dependency means that the field overall operates in a state of financial precarity. Ultimately, this impacts the sustainability and quality of practice in a whole range of ways (explored across this book). An important factor contributing to these challenges is that arts organisations (locally and internationally) have historically been required to produce evidence that aligns with medical model conceptualisations of wellbeing and value and with quantitative 'scientific' approaches to evaluation, such as randomised control trials (Mullen et al. 2021). These approaches are misaligned with arts and wellbeing organisations whose work predominantly addresses the social determinants of health and wellbeing, and who predominantly use qualitative evaluation methods (Tomlinson et al. 2018).

Recent literature proposes that the key to solving these challenges is the development of bespoke evaluation approaches which are more attuned to capturing the complexity of participatory arts practice. It also proposes a need to shift our focus from an almost exclusive emphasis on evidencing *what* outcomes are achieved to consider *how* the arts might work to influence wellbeing (Raw et al. 2013). The conclusion drawn from a scholarly seminar series focused on advancing international arts and wellbeing practice was that the production of theoretically grounded, evidence-informed frameworks which can clearly articulate the aims, methods, theories, and relationships at play in participatory arts settings is needed. Such frameworks should be capable of clearly articulating the unique contribution of arts participation to wellbeing whilst also capturing the characteristics of effective practice settings, and how these differ across contexts (Stickley et al. 2017). They should also be attuned to the values and aspirations of arts organisations as these values can be compromised by misalignment with funder aspirations (Mullen et al. 2021). For example, the dominance of pre-determined outcomes within health policy and practice can limit the ability of AHW practitioners to be participant-led, ultimately reducing their capacity to be responsive to young people's needs and aspirations (Mullen et al. 2021). Our research project set out to respond directly to these concerns by producing a theoretically grounded, evidence-informed practice framework embedded in the specific context of Project X and the diverse perspectives of the project community.

The Project X Research Approach and Theory of Change Workshops

Our research incorporated multiple methods in a staged process. We used a qualitative participatory approach designed to bring together representatives from across the project community to understand Project X from their diverse perspectives and expertise. We adapted a Theory-based Evaluation (TBE) approach designed by Deane et al. (2020) by incorporating arts-based methods. We conducted three participatory focus group workshops with three separate groups who had in-depth knowledge of Project X. In these workshops, we used TBE methods to build a Theory of Change (ToC) for the project. ToC is one approach within the wider family of TBE approaches. The central purpose of ToC is to produce an in-depth understanding about how an initiative is intended to work, and specifically to articulate how the different elements of a social programme (people, activities, context) interact to activate the desired outcomes. This is commonly described as the quest to understand what works, for whom, and in what circumstances (Pawson and Tilley 1997). This ToC can then be used to design an evaluation plan drawing from a range of methods and types of evidence, dependent on the needs of the project.

TBE approaches emerged from recognition that positivist (medical model) approaches are based on linear causal pathways and are limited in their ability to capture the complexity of interactions and interdependencies in social programmes. In TBE change is understood to be complex, unpredictable, non-linear. Participants are not seen as passive recipients of interventions with predictable outcomes, but as active agents whose lived experience plays a significantly influence in what outcomes can be achieved (Galloway 2009). Over the last two to three decades, TBE approaches have become widely used within community and youth programmes and are increasingly of interest in participatory arts settings (Dunphy 2018). Galloway (2009) notes that the appeal of TBE approaches lies both in their ability to articulate the complexity of social settings, and that they lend themselves to qualitative *and* quantitative evaluation approaches. In Project X, we felt that Developmental Evaluation (DE) was the most attuned approach. DE emphasises reflective practice to capture *how* the complexity of interacting elements in social programmes is unfolding in real time. This contrasts to predominant evaluation approaches which focus on *what* outcomes happen at the end (see Quinn Patton et al. 2015). Guided by our ToC, we used DE principles to help us plan our evaluation questions.

We built our ToC Project X over three workshops, each asking questions related to the project vision, intended participants, anticipated outcomes, and the practices, principles, and processes that were critical to the project's effectiveness. We also asked participants to identify the systemic factors that contribute to poor youth mental health and the conditions in the project environment (ecosystem) that might influence its operation.

Workshop 1 involved ten adults, staff and artists from Project X, and representatives from partner health, education, and Kaupapa Māori organisations. We used methods including group discussion, flip charts, and mindmaps to document ideas. We also used Bronfenbrenners' (1979)

Socio-ecological Theory as a useful tool to help us visually map the systemic determinants of youth wellbeing in relation to the nested layers of Bronfenbrenners ecosystem. This process helped us to identify the systemic factors influencing youth wellbeing and which of these factors Project X had the potential to influence.

Workshops 2 and 3 included 11 young people aged 17–23 who had taken part in two Project X pilots. First, participants were asked to respond to research questions by making paintings and collages around a large table. As researchers we made art alongside the group to help collapse power dynamics. Participants articulated their ideas using colourful expressive imagery. An important image that emerged and was developed through the workshops was a tree, which symbolized a person flourishing in a healthy ecosystem. We subsequently framed the theory-building process around the question of what ingredients in Project X grow a healthy tree. We made an outline of a tree on a giant sheet of paper and invited participants to populate it with images, interspersed with conversation to share and unpack ideas. The group made leaves, fruit, worms, gremlins, clouds, and other objects or used words, each articulating different elements of the active ingredients of Project X.

It is impossible to do justice to the findings of our research within this chapter. So, we offer key insights that emphasise the contribution of our process as a tool for 'artful evaluation'. More details of the findings have been published elsewhere (Walls 2024). The three focus groups articulated a shared perception that Project X creates an environment that can positively impact multiple aspects of young people's social and emotional wellbeing. These include therapeutic benefits (relaxation and anxiety reduction) alongside growth of personal and social insights and resources, enabling greater wellbeing and feelings of empowerment and purpose. Participants produced rich and detailed accounts of the active ingredients (critical practices, processes, and principles) at play in Project X, alongside wider environmental factors that also influence outcomes. Many of these were unique to creative processes, the participatory arts context, and facilitation by artists. Collectively they described a complex and dynamic practice ecology that was highly sensitive to interactions between people, place, process, and context. What emerged was a ToC that was highly contextual and embedded in its Pacific context. Foundational te ao Māori (Māori world) concepts were frequently described (by both Māori and non-Māori participants) as being critical to the wellbeing benefits experienced.

Findings were drawn together into a shared Project X ToC. Our ToC summary statement is that:

> Project X offers a safe, mana-enhancing and imaginative space where young people can work creatively together to explore their worlds and grow personal and social resources in support of individual and collective wellbeing. (Walls 2024)

We represented the ToC using images produced during workshops to maintain authenticity and privilege youth voices (Fig. 9.1).

The tree indicates the complex project ecology. Active ingredients (critical practices, processes, principles) are presented in the roots of the tree, feeding healthy growth, with *potential* outcomes represented by leaves and 'blossoms'. Factors influencing the wider ecosystem are summarised in the cloud and gremlin (to the right of the image). Project X involves a highly relational practice aligned with a socio-ecological model of wellbeing grounded in an ethics of care. The critical processes, practices, and principles are grouped into three themes supported by three overarching principles. Each of these themes is overlapping and interdependent with others. Mātauranga Māori (Māori knowledge) concepts and principles are used where these were articulated by research participants. The three critical overarching principles are (1) mana-enhancing, (2) power-sharing, and (3) grounded in young people's worlds. Power-sharing is about collapsing power dynamics, shared decision-making, youth agency, and self-determination. Grounded in young people's worlds acknowledges that wellbeing is shaped systemically by the circumstances of young people's lives. Mana-enhancing draws from the Māori concept mana and refers to the criticality of mana (status, personal power, dignity, and validation) to wellbeing.

Twelve distinct but interconnected practices and processes were identified which were grouped into three themes: (a) relationships, (b) breathing space, and (c) creative and critical exploration. The theme of relationships represents the highly relational nature of the project environment: the building of kinship, special solidarity, support, feelings of validation and belonging, ako (mutual and co-created learning and discovery). The next theme, breathing space (a term used during the workshops), represents spatial elements and includes psychological, physical, social, and conceptual space. This theme includes a space of safety, refuge, and relaxation, transformative space, non-stigmatising setting and

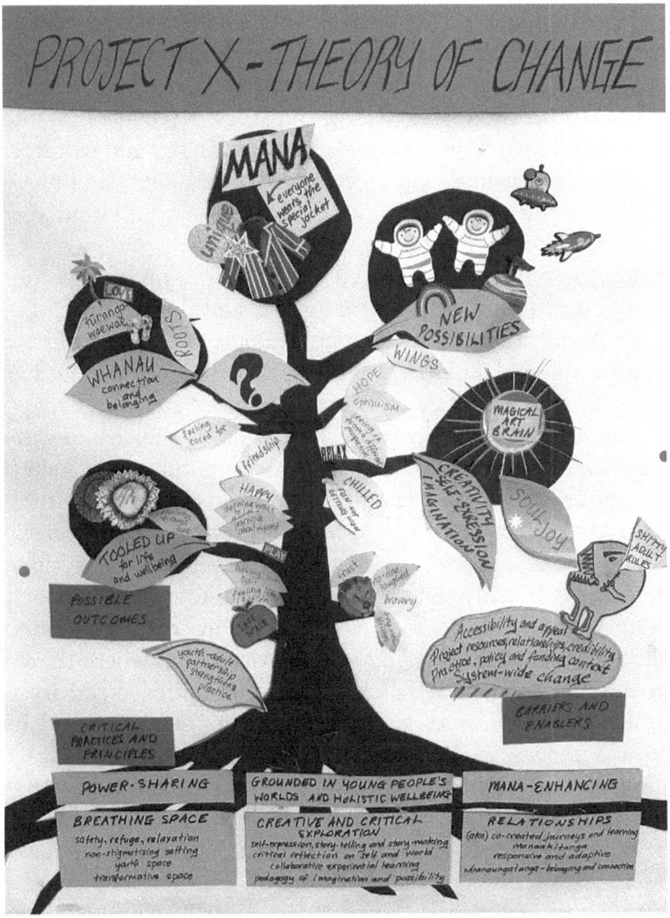

Fig. 9.1 Visual representation of project X ToC. Image credit: Amber Walls (2021)

youth space. These 'spaces' facilitated feelings of safety and freedom from stigma, anxiety, and distress. They enabled freedom to experiment with (potentially transformational) creative and playful processes. They also provided a space for peer connection, mutual support, and collective action, and a space for non-stigmatising engagement with mental health services. The theme creative and critical exploration represents practices and processes that were specifically arts-based (although arts-based processes contribute across all themes). These overlapping practices were defined as self-expression, storytelling and story-making (reframing negative thoughts and life stories), critical reflection on self and world, collaborative experiential learning, and a pedagogy of possibility and imagination (articulating the possibilities enabled by exploratory, unbounded creative, and imaginative processes).

Together, these processes enabled critical reflection on self and world, processes of conscientisation, new pathways, and the building of personal and social resources that helped young people to navigate life, embark on new pathways, and support wellbeing. Key themes to note here were that Project X functioned as a 'breathing space' from everyday experiences of distress for many in the group. Factors which contributed to this space included highly relational practices, a culture of inclusivity in which all unique identities were affirmed, and an environment of manaakitanga (process of caring for others). Restoring mana (authority, worth) and enabling positive identity and self-concept were central to this. Playful experimental arts-based practices also played a key mana-enhancing role by enabling self-expression, 'my own voice', and creating space for non-prescriptive self-directed creativity in an environment where there was no 'right or wrong answer', or failure. This unbounded creativity enabled highly valued experiences of success. For many in the group this environment was experienced as empowering, liberating, and as a catalyst for fuelling passions, 'souljoy', 'imagination', and 'growing wings'. The arts were described by some as taking them to an alternative transformational place and helping them to imagine and then pursue a more positive sense of themselves and their worlds. The arts studio and participatory group practices played a critical role in rebalancing power dynamics by enabling co-creation of artworks, shared decision-making, and self-determined outcomes. Creative experiential practices enabled risk-taking, experimentation, and personal growth in a supportive context. Through reflective arts-based methods participants were able to reframe unhelpful perspectives and develop coping strategies. The need for psychological safety and strengths-based approaches was prominent. Participants highlighted the stark contrast between their experience of Project X and more traditional mental health support services which they associated with experiences of stigma and failure.

Long term possible outcomes for young people have been broadly grouped into five key areas. These outcomes are represented as the outer branches of the tree and organised as whānau (representing feelings of kinship, belonging, and connection to supportive people, histories, and resources); tooled up (with resources for navigating life and wellbeing); mana (achieving potential status, respect, self-belief, self-worth, which for young people is inseparable from self-determination); new possibilities and life stories; plus one group emphasising creativity, self-expression, and imagination. Images drawn from workshops were incorporated into these groupings to represent the ideas and creativity at play. Other outcomes articulated by participants were represented as leaves and 'fruits' in various parts of the tree. These include wings; roots; souljoy; optimism; hope; fun without getting high; magical art brains; self-expression; friendship; finding my voice; taking risks; trying new things; finding purpose; learning about myself, art, life; unsticking negative thought patterns; seeing things differently; new coping strategies and tools for managing wellbeing; experiencing success; and feeling good about myself. These outcomes are deliberately presented as organic leaves or fruits that are dependent on nutrients and a healthy ecosystem to flourish. The outcomes of projects such as these are not mono-directional, and so our ToC also identifies possible outcomes at an organisational level. Reflexive and adaptive practices, shared decision-making, and processes of co-creation and learning not only strengthen responsivity to young people but also facilitate organisational learning and practice innovation.

Barriers and Enablers (environmental factors that also help or hinder the project) are summarised within the cloud under four distinct headings: accessibility and appeal (representing barriers to participation); project resources, relationships, and credibility (including the expertise and aptitudes of facilitators, and relationships within and external to the project that support its functioning); and the practice policy and funding context (emphasising issues impacting sustainability and enabling good practice). System-wide change is used to define wellbeing determinants operating at the macro level which have a significant influence on engagement, outcomes, and operational aspects of the project. Barriers and enablers are accompanied by a gremlin carrying shitty adult rules, representing the pressured, often exclusionary and toxic life environments created by adults.

Next Steps: A Shared Practice Framework for Aotearoa

In the final stage of our research, we conducted an extensive international literature review. In addition to ensuring that our ToC was supported by wider evidence, we were interested to know if it was transferable across settings and if we were able to produce a ToC for other arts and youth wellbeing settings. Our literature search included material spanning multiple 'knowledges' including academic research and evidence, theory, practitioner expertise (e.g. from evaluation reports), lived experience, and mātauranga Māori (indigenous knowledge). We were able to source a wealth of relevant material across multiple disciplinary fields. We privileged peer-reviewed research from credible sources. There was considerable alignment across the literature. Whilst active ingredients were found to be highly contextual and there were some important local distinctions, a common set of active ingredients were identified across international contexts. Many of these were specific to creative processes, mediums, and the participatory arts setting. Overall, a picture of (participatory) arts and youth wellbeing as a highly evolved and dynamic practice with distinct principles and methodologies emerged.

Through a review of existing local practice frameworks, we found that the Project X ToC resonated with Mana Taiohi, the national youth development framework for Aotearoa (Ara Taiohi 2024). We mapped our ToC against Mana Taiohi and produced Mana Taiohi Auaha (Fig. 9.2), a visual depiction of the ways in which creative youth wellbeing practice (grounded in the Project X ToC) can promote young people's development and hauroa (holistic wellbeing). This practice framework is supported by substantial research and evidence and is attuned to the unique local context and mātauranga Māori. Grounded in te ao Māori, Mana Taiohi is framed around the concept of mana. It emphasises whai wāhitanga (young people's active participation, agency, self-determination) and the mana young people have including mauri (life force or spirit), whakapapa (genealogy and history), hononga (connections), and te ao Taiohi (young people's worlds). The framework articulates how youth development can enhance mana through manaakitanga, whai wāhitanga, mātarauranga, and whanaungatanga by articulating the critical practices, processes, and principles as a series of statements in the tree roots. Our refined ToC based on the wider literature review and recognition of alignment with foundational te ao Māori principles states that: collaborative, creative and critical exploration of young people's worlds in an empowering setting activates mana, mauri, storytelling, story-making and resources for life (Walls 2024).

Incorporating Mātauranga Māori: Insights from Borni

It's vital to understand that te ao Māori, our Māori Tikanga, our processes and our concepts are multifaceted. We are not a homogenous people; therefore, these processes are not easily translated (directly) for non-Māori. There are intricate differences in how we navigate the world dependent on our ancestral connections, which part of the country we connect to, whether we are from an urbanised or rural background and most definitely whether we are enmeshed in the traditional practices of our people or not.

Any piece of work that uses guidance from Māori concepts and processes needs to be done with respect and due diligence. Frameworks such as Te Whare Tapa Whā by Matua Mason Durie (Rochford 2004) and Mana Taiohi Auaha (Walls 2024) have been created with forethought and strict process, and are either created by and/or with the input of respected Māori leaders, Kaumatua (elders), Kaiako (teachers), and Kaiārahi (guides/consultants). These frameworks allow non-Māori to be guided in how to use approaches that are for many Māori, innate. They provide a gateway of understanding to the specificities and richness of Māori practices.

Part of the richness of Te Reo Māori (Māori language) is that many of our words have different meanings depending on the context being used. Mana Taiohi (Ara Taiohi 2024) is accompanied by incredibly strong resource material. Each component is broken down so that you understand how the framework aligns with a specific concept and is paired with an appropriate Whakatauki (Māori proverb). It has been translated and broken down by experts specifically for this development framework so there is no mistaking the authors' purpose. Even with these framework tools, it is still necessary to seek guidance and walk alongside someone who believes in your mahi (work), and trusts that your engagement with Māori principles run deeper than a box ticking exercise. The needs of this project sat comfortably in my (Borni) wheelhouse as Kaiārahi. Any work that needed deeper attention we took to Kaumatua and trusted advisors. As Kaiārahi, the main role was to help discover how the project

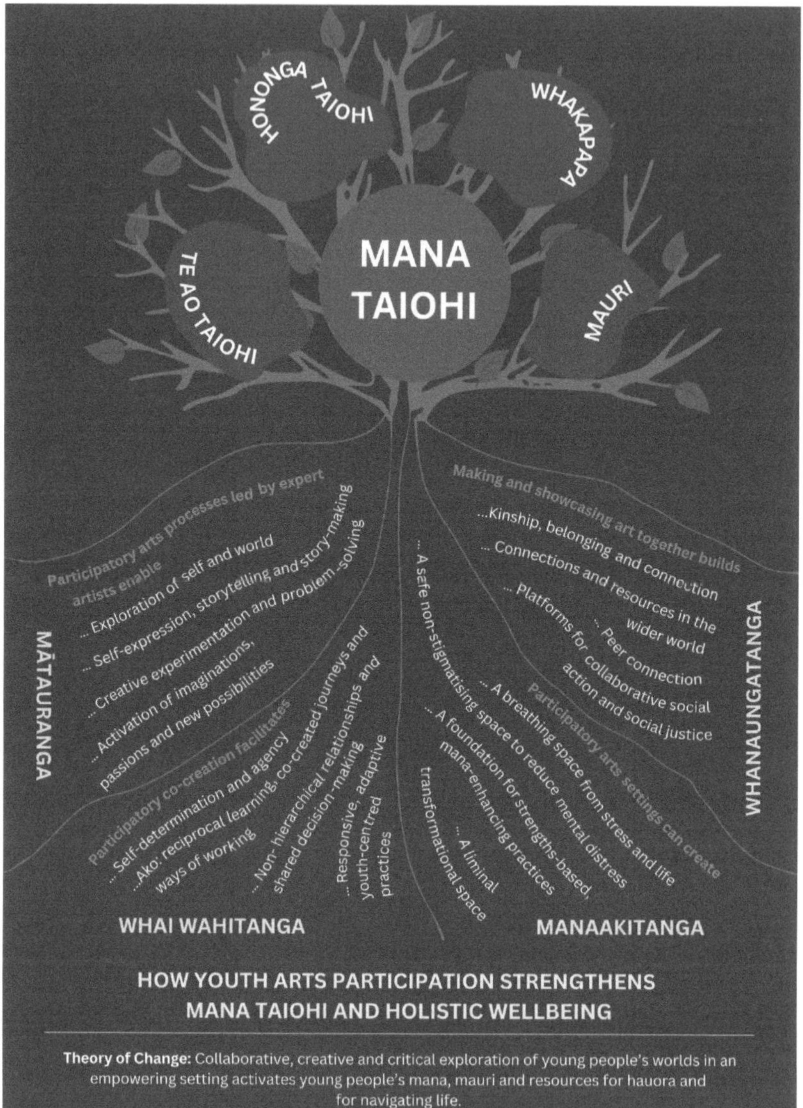

Fig. 9.2 Mana Taiohi Auaha: A creative youth wellbeing practice framework for Aotearoa. Designed by: Asha Munn (2023)

authentically aligned with the concepts and methodologies of the chosen development framework, that the engagement was respectful and transparent and that there was accountability where and if needed throughout the whole process. Amber and I have worked alongside each other for more than seven years as advocates for wellness and bettering the lives of communities across Aotearoa. We have built trust and mutual respect, giving us an easeful dialogue. This allowed us to collaborate clearly on the approach for the ToC ensuring that these tools truly supported the needs of the participatory process of Project X.

Key Insights and Implications for 'Artful Evaluation'

The TBE process we used to develop the ToC for Project X was an excellent and highly replicable approach that can be adapted across arts and wellbeing settings to support 'artful evaluation'. The process enabled us to clearly articulate a rich, culturally embedded understanding of Project X grounded in lived experience, research, evidence, and multiple knowledge systems. It provided a solid foundation to develop shared understanding between project staff, participants, and funders about the possibilities (and limits) of our project. Ultimately, it informed design of meaningful evaluation. Although our research benefited from a university research partnership, the key elements could (and have) been used in other participatory project settings in less resource-intensive ways. In this section, we share three key insights about aspects of our process that were particularly valuable to us, and we think could inform others.

Firstly, the theory-building process was highly collaborative and enabled diverse perspectives and marginalised voices to be heard and incorporated. The ToC process facilitated a collaborative process; however, inclusivity was particularly supported by use of visual arts-based research methods (ABR). ABR methods can provide powerful and accessible languages to express complex ideas and enable rich descriptions of experience and emotions (Leavy 2015). They can be an especially powerful medium to facilitate voices which are marginalised and not heard (Parsons and Boydell 2012). Most participants in our workshops experienced social anxiety and would have struggled to engage with a traditional focus group. However, all participants engaged meaningfully in sharing their perspectives through creative media, and some reported that the arts were the only way they felt able to express themselves. We found that the process of making visual images gave participants time to reflect deeply, respond at their own pace and offer insights in ways that felt safe and self-directed. Everyone making images together created a collaborative space, helped to blur boundaries and rebalance power dynamics between researcher and participant. We incorporated images produced during workshops into our final ToC visual representation. This resulted in a unique visual tool which represents youth perspectives in an authentic and compelling way. The visual representation has been used to powerfully articulate the principles, practices, and possibilities offered by Project X amongst young people, project staff, partner organisations, and funders.

We also found that, contrary to critique in arts literature that ToC is a reductionist method that will stifle the dynamism and potential of participatory arts (Dunphy 2018), ToC methodology enabled us to articulate a rich, highly distinct, and dynamic project ecology. The staged process of questioning different aspects of the project challenged assumptions, advanced our thinking, and introduced important questions related to evaluation and impacts. Introducing the concept of change was particularly effective in generating discussion about 'what change, and whose idea of change is privileged'. Our use of ecological frameworks and metaphors supported thinking about the systemic drivers of wellbeing, and this prompted important discussion about the limits of an individually focused programme such as Project X. In summary, ToC methodology lent itself well to an in-depth, challenging and meaningful process of critical inquiry. This culminated in an understanding that wellbeing is subjective and diverse, and that Project X is complex, precarious, political, socially, culturally, and environmentally contextual. As noted earlier, TBE emerged from recognition that positivist (medical model) approaches are limited in their ability to capture the complexity of interactions and interdependencies in social programmes. Our research highlighted that settings such as Project X require evaluation of the complex relationships, practices, and processes at play to enable ongoing reflection adaptation and responsivity. As noted earlier, we used a Developmental Evaluation (DE) evaluation approach. Guided by the Project X ToC (critical processes, practices, principles), we used DE principles to help us review how well we were meeting our intentions, incorporating 'feedback loops' to capture different perspectives throughout the project. Our evaluation approach shifted from a focus on what *outcomes* individuals might report at the end of their participation, to how well we were creating the *conditions* that would support participants to navigate life and strengthen wellbeing in ways that they valued.

Finally, our research revealed a highly distinct practice methodology through which some arts-based approaches can uniquely activate wellbeing outcomes. These outcomes align with the wellbeing aspirations of participants involved in our study, and those stated by young people in wider literature (Fleming et al. 2020). However, they are not aligned with the goals of predominant mental health support services and associated evaluation models. Examples include descriptions of the ways in which creative experimentation, imagination and risk-taking in Project X offered a breathing space from stress, enabled feelings of liberation and hope, and new life stories to emerge. Our ToC indicates that arts-based approaches are likely to support different goals to clinically-focused health services. Indeed, our ToC is more aligned with empowerment and social justice practices and the positive youth development field. This mismatch highlights the potential of arts-based approaches to address gaps in current practice, but also further signals the need for bespoke practice and evaluation frameworks that can fully capture this potential. Consistent with contemporary literature on advancing youth mental health practice in Aotearoa (see Poulton et al. 2020) we believe this insight also demonstrates the importance of meaningful engagement with participants to shape our understanding of how we might support their wellbeing. Notably, in addition to laying foundations for an evaluation framework, our ToC workshops also functioned as a co-design of Project X. The research workshops resulted in a redesign of Project X including the establishment of a new hub focused on youth-led creative programmes and social action (on the systemic determinants of youth wellbeing). The hub was conceived and led by participants in our ToC research project and demonstrates a further contribution of the study to both organisational and individual wellbeing.[2]

References

Anae, Melani, Helen Moewaka Barnes, Tim McCreanor, and Peter Watson. 2002. *Towards promoting youth mental health in Aotearoa/New Zealand: Holistic 'houses' of health. International Journal of Mental Health Promotion 4(2): 5–14.*

[2] For a more in-depth understanding of this research project see Walls (2024).

Ara Taiohi. *Mana Taiohi*. Available online: https://arataiohi.org.nz/mana-taiohi/. Accessed 1 Oct 2024.

Bronfenbrenner, Urie. 1979. The Ecology of Human Development: Experiments in Nature and Design. Cambridge, MA: Harvard University Press.

Critical Research Unit in Applied Theatre. 2019. Creative Practice for Youth Wellbeing in Aotearoa. The University of Auckland.

Deane, Kelsey, Hilary Dutton, and Pat Bullen. 2020. Theoretically integrative evaluation practice: A step-by step overview of an eclectic evaluation design process. Evaluation 26(1): 98–118.

Dunphy, Kim. 2018. Theorising arts participation as a social change mechanism. In Lee-Bartleet, B. and Higgins, L. (eds) The Oxford Handbook of Community Music. Oxford: Oxford Academic.

Easwaran, Kamala, Lakshmi Narasimhan, Anussha Murali, Deepika Easwaran, Tasneem Raja, and Yog Japee. 2021. Why art matters for youth mental health: A youth led participatory insight analysis. Economic Behavior and Organisation 27(1): 35–47.

Fleming, Terry, Jude Ball, Kristy Kang, Kylie Sutcliffe., Lambert, Michelle., Roshini Peiris-John, and Terryann Clark. 2020. Youth19: Youth Voice Brief. The Youth19 Research Group. Wellington https://static1.squarespace.com/static/5bdbb75ccef37259122e59aa/t/5f3394a2654885030c051243/1597215912482/Youth19+Youth+Voice+Brief.pdf. Accessed 15 Aug 2024.

Freebody, Kelly, Molly Mullen, Amber Walls, and Peter O'Connor. 2019. Who is Responsible? Neoliberal discourses of well-being in Australia and New Zealand. Drama Australia Journal 42(2): 139–153.

Galloway, Susan. 2009. Theory-based evaluation and the social impact of the arts. Cultural Trends. 18(2): 125–148.

Leavy, Patricia. 2015. *Method meets art: Arts-based research practice*. New York: Guilford Press.

Mullen, Molly, Amber Walls, Maria Ahmad, Peter O'Connor. 2021. Resourcing the Arts for Youth Well-Being: challenges in Aotearoa. Arts & Health. 15(1): 71–85.

Parsons, Janet, and Katherine Boydell. 2012. Arts-based research and knowledge translation: Some key concerns for health-care professionals. Journal of Interprofessional Care. 26(3): 170–172.

Pawson, Ray, and Nicholas Tilley. (1997) Realistic Evaluation. London: SAGE.

Poulton, Richie, Peter Gluckman, Rochelle Menzies, Anne Bardsley, Tracey McIntosh, and Monique Faleafa. 2020. Protecting and Promoting Mental Wellbeing: Beyond COVID-19. Koi Tū: The Centre for Informed Futures. https://informedfutures.org/wp-content/uploads/Protecting-and-Promoting-Mental-Wellbeing.pdf Accessed 5 August 2024.

Quinn Patton, Michael, Kate McKegg and Nan Wehipeihana. (2015) Developmental Evaluation Exemplars: Principles in Practice. New York: Guilford Press.

Raw, Anni, and Ana Rosa Mantecón. (2013). Evidence of a transnational arts and health practice methodology? A contextual framing for comparative community-based participatory arts practice in the UK and Mexico. Arts Health. 5(3), 216–229.

Rochford, Tim. 2004. Whare Tapa Wha: A Māori Model of a Unified Theory of Health. The Journal of Primary Prevention. 25: 41–57.

Stickley, Theo, Hester Parr, Hester Parr, Sarah Atkinson, Norma Daykin, Stephen Clift, Tia De Nora, Sue Hacking, Paul M Camic, Tim Joss, Mike White, and Susan J Hogan. 2017. Arts, health and wellbeing: Arts, health and wellbeing: Reflections on a national seminar series and building a UK research network. Arts & Health. 9(1): 14–25.

Tomlinson, Alan, Jack Lane, Guy Julier, Lily Grigsby-Duffy, Annette Payne, Louise Mansfield, Tess Kay, Alistair John, Catherine Meads, Norma Daykin, Kerry Ball, Christine Tapson, Paul Dolan, Stefano Testoni, and Christina Victor. 2018. A systematic review of the subjective wellbeing outcomes of engaging with visual arts for adults with diagnosed mental health conditions. What Works Centre for Wellbeing. https://aru.figshare.com/articles/report/A_systematic_review_of_the_subjective_wellbeing_outcomes_of_engaging_with_visual_arts_for_adults_working-age_15-64_years_with_diagnosed_mental_health_conditions/23783646?file=41717517. Accessed 1 October 2023.

Walls, Amber. 2024. Activating the arts for youth wellbeing in Aotearoa: Practices, principles and possibilities. Dissertation, University of Auckland.

CHAPTER 10

Participatory Songwriting as Evaluative Research: Learning from Adolescent Experiences of Voice and Voicelessness

Gillian Howell

Introduction

Article 12 of the United Nations Convention on the Rights of the Child (UNCRC) enshrines rights of children to "express [their] views freely on all matters affecting [them]" and for those views to be "given due weight in accordance with [their] age and maturity" (United Nations 1989, art. 12). These obligations of ensuring space for the free expression of views and the giving of due weight to what is expressed, places equal emphasis on the processes of voicing and listening. Arts-based research and evaluation approaches can be valuable tools in fulfilling this dual mandate with adolescents, offering innovative ways to amplify their voices via multiple

G. Howell (✉)
School of Humanities, Creative Industries and Social Sciences, University of Newcastle, Newcastle, Australia
e-mail: ghowell@unimelb.edu.au; gillian@gillianhowell.com.au

Faculty of Fine Arts and Music, University of Melbourne, Melbourne, VIC, Australia

M. Mullen et al. (eds.), *Artful Evaluation for Creative Health and Wellbeing*, New Directions in Cultural Policy Research,
https://doi.org/10.1007/978-3-032-17063-7_10

platforms, connect with listeners on an emotional and empathetic level, and inspire decision-makers to move beyond traditional, often decontextualised interpretations of research data. This chapter is about how I used songwriting within a humanitarian aid and development project as a research method to centre adolescent voices and position young people as co-producers of knowledge.

As other chapters in this anthology attest, an artful approach to research and evaluation can bring both experiential and empirical benefits, and offer a way to circumvent the adult-centric power structures and epistemologies of many conventional research approaches. These can often reinforce the very exclusions they seek to understand (Nguyen et al. 2021). The participatory songwriting presented here sought to provide a meaningful, engaging modality for adolescents to "name their world", which Freire describes as the process of critically identifying and analysing the social realities that shape one's life (Freire 2000/1970, 88). As they progress through the songwriting process, participants narrate their experiences and engage in the co-production of knowledge, producing not just rich narrative data but research outputs—in the form of original songs—that can inform programme adaptation and wider dissemination. The methodology aligns well with a developmental evaluation approach, supporting learning-oriented goals of problem identification, concept development, iterative testing of new ideas, and the real-time integration of new information in complex, emergent settings (Patton 2011).

The chapter draws on my experiences co-delivering this methodology with Syrian, Palestinian, and Jordanian adolescents aged 14–19 in Jordan, Lebanon, and Türkiye. It addresses the question: how might participatory songwriting be used as a research method that centres voice and positions adolescent participants as co-producers of knowledge in humanitarian contexts? The chapter outlines the research context, explores ethical considerations, and provides a detailed description of the methodology. I conclude that participatory songwriting offers an important arts-based research method in complex settings. It offers a relational, non-extractive, youth-centred approach that supports ethical engagement and collaborative meaning-making through shared creative expression.

The Research Context: Adolescents Affected by War, Violence, and Displacement

The methodology was developed and put into practice following a research commission that I received from Save the Children International's Middle East and Eastern Europe regional office (henceforth SCI-ME) in 2021.[1] SCI-ME was redeveloping its adolescent programme delivery in the region (which includes country offices in Jordan, Lebanon, Türkiye, Egypt, and Iraq), a process that involved research with their constituents to identify key themes and concerns. Earlier SCI-ME research (Mason 2019) had identified the shocking levels of violence that refugees and displaced adolescents in these countries were navigating in the home, in schools, and workplaces, and through harmful and discriminatory state policies and cultural norms towards refugees and displaced people. The previous research highlighted that these multiple forms of violence exacerbated adolescents' feelings of voicelessness and disempowerment, creating complex barriers to the realisation of adolescent goals of personal growth and opportunities for meaningful civic participation. The new SCI-ME commissioned research aimed to explore these adolescent experiences of voice and voicelessness using arts-based methods, as these had been proven to be highly effective in the 2019 research. They also wanted to enhance local staff capacity to use arts-based research methods in their ongoing monitoring, evaluation, and learning. They selected my proposal to deliver the research through participatory songwriting through an international tender process.[2]

This project integrated my two decades of work as a music facilitator and researcher with war-impacted adolescents in Australia, Bosnia-Herzegovina, and Georgia, and with First Nations youth in Australia into a participatory research methodology. Having led several evaluations for cultural organisations, I recognised participatory songwriting's potential to amplify adolescent voices in a format meaningful to them that is also

[1] Save the Children International is a global aid and development organisation dedicated to protecting and supporting children in need.

[2] The full study had four research questions: (1) How do adolescents affected by conflict and violence in Lebanon, Jordan, and Türkiye experience 'voice' and collective power? (2) What are the barriers (such as power structures, social and gender norms) that limit the agency of adolescents? (3) How do their experiences of violence influence voice, activism, and engagement with power structures? (4) What are the opportunities for nurturing greater civic engagement, voice, and agency among this cohort?

compelling for decision-makers. This approach addressed the UNCRC's mandate for children's voices to be both heard and given due weight, offering a powerful tool for engagement beyond traditional speech or text-based methods.

It is unusual to see a call for tenders for *arts-based* research in the global development sector. Artistic activity has long been used to support humanitarian and development goals; however, global development endeavours tend to be "driven, designed, implemented, and evaluated via linear models based on cold, rational logic" (Ware et al. 2025, 4). Participatory arts-based research (PABR), though gaining modest recognition within development research, remains far from being embraced as a core methodology in the sector. In contrast, other fields have increasingly legitimised PABR for its ability to amplify marginalised voices, explore sensitive topics through metaphor and symbol, and generate evidence that resonates experientially as well as empirically (Leavy 2020). As an emerging approach in development settings, PABR has shown particular promise with children and young people who have experienced adversity, including war-impacted children and young people, (Green and Denov 2019; Pavarini et al. 2021) and girls with disabilities in Vietnam (Nguyen et al. 2021). But despite music's ubiquity within youth cultures and relevance to key development priorities—such as social-emotional wellbeing, youth participation, and increasing research participant agency—music and songwriting remain underutilised within PABR and are the least reported in systematic and scoping reviews of arts-based research publications (Boydell et al. 2016; Coemans and Hannes 2017; Leavy 2020, 132).

Given the low representation of music-making in PABR, what is known about music-based approaches to evaluation and research comes largely from music therapy. This literature presents participatory songwriting as a strengths-based approach that can support youth to explore sensitive topics metaphorically, reframe personal narratives, and assume authority as experts in their lives (Bolger 2015; Fairchild and McFerran 2019). These accounts show the potential for participatory songwriting to position young people in research as "full actors with diverse needs" (Singh et al. 2023, 2), challenging the pervasive emphasis in humanitarian research on risk and vulnerability and shifting it to one of strength and competencies.

The NGO that commissioned me, referred to here as SCI-ME, was curious about the potential of music-based methods in participatory research, given that the previous research conducted in 2019 had used visual arts and theatre methods, and local staff were eager to expand their methodological toolkit for in-house research. They recognised music's prominence in young people's expressive lives, and that songwriting could allow participants to explore the theme of voice through their own vocal expression. This complementarity presented the potential to generate rich text-based data through lyrics, with finished songs giving participants a chance to name and talk back to the silencing forces in their lives.

Conceptual Framework: A Socio-Ecological Model of Adolescent Voice

Conceptually, "voice" was understood as the capacity to vocalise thoughts, ideas and experiences, contribute one's voice on matters of concern, and situate oneself relationally within broader structures and systems (Couldry 2010). Embracing Cavarero's (2005) notion of voice representing uniqueness in both individual and collective expressions, this conceptualisation aligned with de Quadros and Amrein's view of "the voice identify[ing]...the self relationally and politically" (2022, 77). Thus, voice served as a metaphor for considering experiences of power and influence in social settings (Juffermans and Van der Aa 2013).

Conceptualising voice as socially and politically grounded suggested that an ecological approach to the study would be valuable, prompting the development of a socio-ecological model (SEM) of adolescent voice specific to the Middle East context. Bronfenbrenner's socio-ecological model of human development (1977) was an important starting point. Bronfenbrenner's model conceptualises human development as a complex interplay between multiple systems (or layers) of influence, from systems of direct interaction, such as the family, workplace, or school, to those of increasingly indirect influence (such as cultural values, structural norms, and historical events). I created a bespoke model that would specify the systems of influence for the study participants, most of whom were displaced and living in large settlements for Palestinian and Syrian refugees in Jordan, Lebanon, and Türkiye. I used the first-person quotes and findings in SCI-ME's 2019 research report to identify the dominant social structures impacting adolescent voice in these contexts (Mason 2019), developing these into a context-specific SEM (Fig. 10.1). SCI-ME staff reviewed the bespoke model and confirmed its salience prior to me finalising the research design, and the SEM was then used to prompt reflections and narratives in the songwriting workshops.

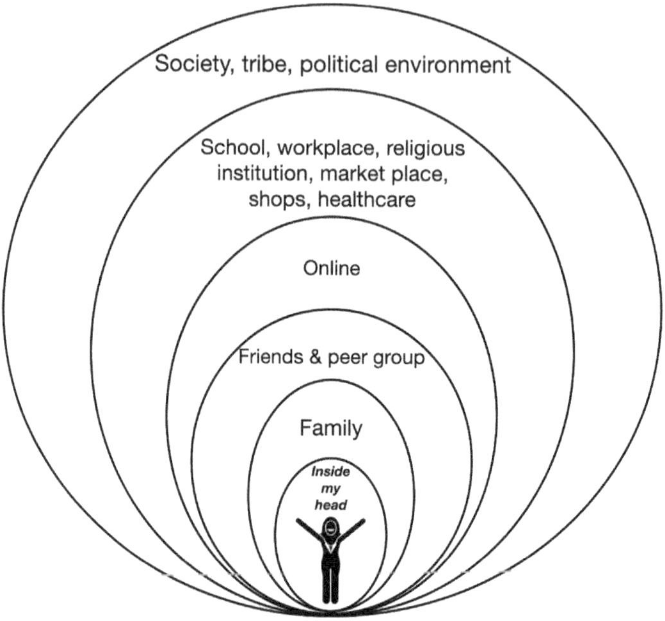

Fig. 10.1 Socio-ecological model [SEM] for "voice" in the lives of adolescents affected by conflict in Lebanon, Jordan, and Türkiye. Developed by G. Howell, based on Bronfenbrenner (1977)

Project Preparations and Delivery

This international research project, conducted in November–December 2021, navigated the challenges of COVID-19 travel restrictions and border closures. Unable to leave Australia, I coordinated the project remotely from Melbourne, leveraging my international networks to recruit an experienced Arabic-speaking musician based in the region. Ameen Mokdad, an Iraqi musician, composer, and poet with firsthand experience of conflict and displacement, was selected to facilitate the song-writing workshops. Ameen and I collaborated via Zoom to develop the workshop approach, with Ameen completing online training in research ethics, child protection, and risk management. At SCI-ME's request,

Ameen piloted the methodology at the Tarkib Contemporary Art Institute in Baghdad, leading a one-day workshop with adolescents and young adults.

The SCI-ME regional office coordinated with country offices in Lebanon, Jordan, and Türkiye to select workshop sites and local partners. Each workshop was led by Ameen, supported by a team of local staff from SCI country offices and partner organisations. We provided comprehensive training for local staff, beginning with two days of online sessions led by me, covering the research approach, ethics, recruitment, and inclusion. Ameen then conducted a one-day, in-person workshop at each site, introducing participatory songwriting-as-research. Staff explored their own experiences of voice and voicelessness, creating shared songs. These experiential sessions built staff confidence in the research approach, particularly for those more familiar with conventional research methods.

In total, 11 workshops were held across the three countries: four in Lebanon, five in Jordan, and two in Türkiye. Each 3- to 4.5-hour session took place in refugee camps and community centres supporting displaced and disadvantaged communities. Partner staff recruited 110 adolescent participants aged 14–19 years,[3] all currently involved in local programmes for adolescents.[4] The sample included 63 Syrian refugees, 30 Jordanians, and 17 Palestinians. Workshops were conducted in Arabic, with staff taking detailed notes on verbal and non-verbal interactions. These notes, along with song lyrics, were translated into English and uploaded to a shared online folder. Ameen and I held daily debriefing calls to review and clarify the data. The project dataset comprised workshop notes, debrief notes, song lyrics, audio recordings, and participant drawings. We implemented a two-tiered consent process: first, for study participation (obtained from parents/caregivers or participants over 18), and second, for sharing the finished songs with wider audiences. The latter was discussed with participants at the end of each workshop, affirming their ownership of the co-created songs and the right to determine their

[3] SCI defines adolescence as the transition from childhood to adulthood, a life-stage that is contextual and influenced by many factors. For its adolescent service provision, SCI has adopted the age-based definition used by UNICEF and the World Health Organisation of adolescence as between 10 and 19 years of age. SCI-ME specified the target age range for this research as 14–19 years.

[4] Programmes for adolescents include Life Skills, Mental Health and Psychosocial Support, and football training, among others.

dissemination. This extensive preparation set the stage for the workshops, which began in Lebanon. The following section details the methodology, highlighting the interplay between creative process and qualitative inquiry.

Participatory Songwriting Research Method

The research design took as its starting point a collaborative songwriting research method from music therapy (Fairchild and McFerran 2019). That method involved children as co-constructors of knowledge via songwriting in response to a guiding research question. My adaptations were to use the bespoke socio-ecological model (SEM) to guide brainstorming and storytelling, and through the development of additional participatory analysis steps in the songwriting workshops. Like Fairchild and McFerran, I found that the creative stages for participatory songwriting—generation of ideas through storytelling and narrative, identification of emergent themes, collation of related ideas, distillation of these into concise forms suitable for song lyrics, and song finalising and recording—mirrored the respective research steps of data generation, data analysis, and presentation of findings, but in an arts-led way (Fairchild and McFerran 2019, 94).

Step One: Warming Up and Introducing the Conceptual Framing for Voice

Each workshop began with ice-breaker activities and warm-up games to set a relaxed and playful tone for the workshop, build an encouraging environment, stimulate creative thinking, and reduce participant self-consciousness. Following the warm-up, Ameen showed the participants a diagram of the socio-ecological model for adolescent voice and invited them to reflect on the ways they modified their voice and vocal expression in the different spaces and relationships in their lives.

Step Two: Sharing Stories of Voice Experiences

Ameen asked the participants to consider the spaces and relationships represented in the SEM in which their voices felt strongest, and the spaces where their voices felt most quiet, or where they felt voiceless. Some groups also considered a sixth dimension, that of the *internal* voice. They took turns sharing stories about their experiences, with the project staff recording these in writing, aiming to remain true to the speaker's actual words. Starting with stories of strong voices enabled the adolescents to move gradually from positive experiences towards stories depicting feelings of disempowerment and exclusion. The participants were not obliged to share their "voice" experience in all five spaces, leaving them in control of the stories they shared.

Step Three: Developing Conceptual Labels

At the conclusion of each shared story, the storyteller chose a descriptive or metaphoric label that captured the experience of "voice" depicted in the story and wrote it on a piece of coloured paper (Fig. 10.2). The assigning of labels by the storytellers was the first analytic layer and ensured the creative process foregrounded the adolescents' ideas and meaning-making ahead of researcher interpretations of what they shared. The creation of these labels invited the storytellers—often assisted by others in the group—to "think up" from the raw data and begin to organise their experiences into conceptual categories.

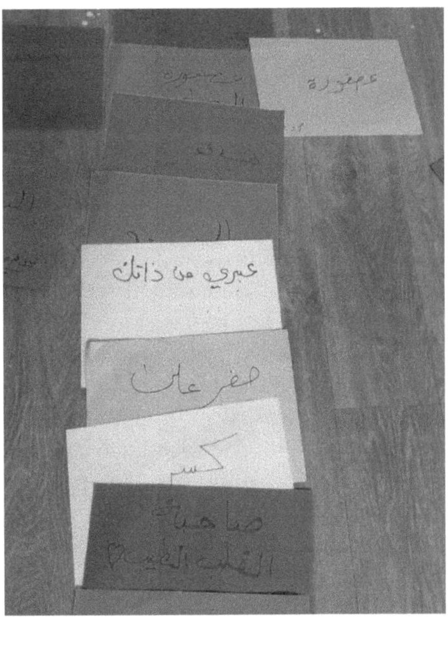

Fig. 10.2 Descriptive and metaphoric labels chosen at a workshop in Jordan. Image by A. Mokdad

Metaphor development was a purposeful part of this process. Metaphors can provide useful conceptual language in creative work and research, making abstract concepts more concrete, or offering a way to reflect on experiences through different perspectives (Ware 2022). They can facilitate communication of difficult experiences in ambiguous or indirect ways and allow multiple interpretations to co-exist. In this project, metaphors emerged as powerful vehicles for conveying the intensity of affect and embodied experiences. These metaphors—such as a closed box, a caged bird, a bright light in the distance, or a silent lion—functioned as evocative knowledge translation tools, bridging the gap between the lived experiences of adolescents and their audiences.

Each metaphor carried a rich tapestry of meaning, emotion, and sensory experience. For example, one girl (16–19 years, Lebanon) chose the metaphor of a white gazelle "because it is endangered and needs protection". By likening her voice to an endangered species, she conveyed the fragility of her right to be heard and the urgent need for protection and conservation of that right. Metaphors, therefore, served as conduits for emotional resonance and empathetic understanding. They allowed the adolescents to communicate complex, often painful realities, in ways that were both personally meaningful and universally comprehensible, making their lived experiences more knowable and potentially more actionable to others.

Step Four: Co-Creating a Narrative Arc

At the conclusion of the story-sharing and metaphor development, the group explored the relationships between the labels they had amassed and collated them thematically. Ameen then asked the group to create a single narrative "arc" that could incorporate all these words and metaphors. The narrative became the basis for a group song. This step represents the second analytic layer, where the group works collectively to thematise and condense their conceptual categories into a higher-order interpretive narrative or allegory.

Separate pages for each analytic label made the process more interactive; by moving pages around, participants were making their thought processes and decision-making visible, helping to prompt new ideas in others, which facilitated a collective analysis process. The workshop team documented the group's decision-making and Ameen helped them organise their narrative into lyrics. To illustrate this process, the metaphors for the song The Jungle (composed by boys, 16–19 years, Burj al Barajneh, Beirut, Lebanon) were: responsible, home, careful, annoying voice, silent voice, wolf, jungle, lion, tiger, conflict, war, we, problems. The lyrics below show their integration into a collective narrative:

I am careful in the jungle.
Like a fox warning of death.
Responsible for my flock.
The cries of the dead bother me.
And people cry without a sound.
And leave my land without a sound.
Because of a war between a lion and a tiger.
We argue—with whom should we run?
With a responsible lion?
Or a rebellious tiger?
And our fear grows.
Between hunger and thirst,
Disease and poverty,
War and security.
And the injustice is increasing.
Day after day.
I live in oppression and in war.
And I am lost, confused.
Like a whirlpool swirling and swirling.
Song: The Jungle, by boys, 16–19 years, Lebanon

Through this step, the narrative arc served as a dramaturgical device that facilitated multiple forms of connection. It brought together participants' diverse experiences across different relational domains, encouraging shared understanding and deepening group cohesion. At the same time, it threaded the metaphors into a more cohesive whole, enriching their meanings through juxtaposition and layering. The resulting song lyrics served as a compact and powerful form of research translation, articulating the adolescents' experiences of voice with broader audiences.

Step Five: Composing and Recording the Song

Ameen then helped the group to create a melody and rhythm for their words, accompanying them on the violin. The songs were short (most were under a minute long) and varied in musical styles, from folk-inflected melodies to rap, to spoken word. The workshop participants rehearsed their song together and recorded it (Fig. 10.3). Those with phones were able to transfer their recorded song to their phones before the workshop ended. The hope was to include all the songs from the project in a digital album that could be shared with all the participants and that they could share with others. But this was not assumed; instead, Ameen and the workshop staff invited the participants to discuss the possible audiences (including the other adolescent songwriters taking part in the research, SCI-ME, audiences in conference presentations, and making the album full open access) and reach agreement on the scope of their song's distribution. Each group proved eager to share their song, and the album was made freely available to all.[5]

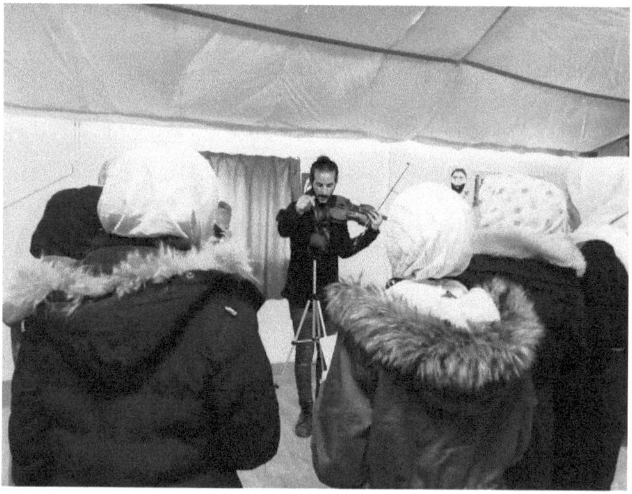

Fig. 10.3 Girls aged 14–17 years in Za'atari Camp record their song. Image by A. Mokdad

[5] The album and lyrics can be accessed here: https://soundcloud.com/user-914416312/sets/silent-lions-songs-by-adolescents-affected-by-war-and-violent-conflict.

Step Six: Reflecting and Drawing Together

At the conclusion of the music-making activities in Lebanon and Türkiye, the participants reflected on their workshop experience and voice narratives through drawing (time pressures meant that this activity did not happen in Jordan). Ameen provided high-quality paper and richly pigmented markers and pastels to ensure a sensory, aesthetically satisfying experience. Drawing gave the participants time to process the songwriting workshop experience while still in the shared space. It also gave the workshops a "soft" ending, allowing time for informal conversations with each other and the workshop team and to listen to their song recording a few more times. For the research, the artworks offered a visual depiction of the participants' voice experiences and formed part of the dataset for analysis and triangulation.

Step Seven: Compilation of Data

Given the project's time constraints, we chose not to use video or audio recordings, which would have required extensive translation and transcription. Instead, we implemented a robust data compilation protocol. This involved two team members taking concurrent notes during each workshop, followed by a group debrief immediately after. During these debriefs, the team used their notes to stimulate recall, collaboratively refining and expanding the documentation with additional details about participants' stories and words. Local staff provided valuable contextual information, linking participants' narratives to current community issues and debates. This process ensured that the final documentation reflected a comprehensive and consensual account of the workshop. Following each session, the notes were consolidated into a single document, translated into English, and securely uploaded to an encrypted cloud-based drive for subsequent cross-case analysis.

Step Eight: Cross-Case Analysis

The 11 workshops and three in-person staff training days took place over a 20-day period. Following its conclusion, I analysed the full dataset, comparing adolescent voice experiences across cases and according to gender, age, and geographic location within each of the "systems of influence" of the SEM. I produced a detailed report in English for SCI-ME,[6] accompanied by a webinar summarising the findings and recommendations for global SCI-ME staff. The findings can only be briefly summarised here. The study revealed a complex landscape of adolescent voice experiences across all age groups and sites. Overwhelmingly, adolescents reported feeling voiceless, leading to a range of emotional responses including indignation, frustration, and anger. Some, particularly older girls aged 16–19, expressed fear and despair as they perceived their vocal space rapidly shrinking. In contrast, boys generally experienced expanding vocal space as they aged, reflecting prevailing cultural norms and the increased restrictions on girls' autonomy in displacement contexts (Jones et al. 2021). Participants painted a challenging picture of their journey to adulthood within highly hierarchical social structures. They described environments characterised by lawlessness and lack of accountability, where speaking up often carried significant risks. This led many to self-censor or carefully select moments to express themselves.

Experiences varied across different social systems. The family emerged as a complex site, with 45% of participants reporting it as a space where they had a strong voice, while 30% described it as a site of silencing. Schools and workplaces elicited similarly ambivalent responses. Online spaces were generally perceived as silencing, though interestingly, some older girls found these to be their only avenue for agency and purpose. One participant, a 16–19-year-old girl from Lebanon, shared:

> I have five teams whom I train in leadership skills. I use social media to give my workshops, but I would prefer to meet face-to-face. [...] I have no choice because my family doesn't allow me to leave the house a lot. So, I have strong voice in the community but not at home. (Girl, 16–19 years, Lebanon)

Others highlighted the risks of online expression, citing incidents where a series of humorous memes shared among the Syrian refugee community led to deportations of Syrian refugees in Türkiye. Alongside these challenges, the cross-case analysis identified vital pockets of vocal freedom and

[6] The full report is available from https://findanexpert.unimelb.edu.au/scholarlywork/1679772-silent-lions%2D%2Dexperiences-of-voice-and-collective-power-among-adolescent-girls-and-boys-affected-by-conflict-and-violence-in-lebanon%2D%2Djordan%2D%2Dand-turkey.

personal growth. These sites of agency and initiative informed the development of seven recommendations to SCI-ME for its future adolescent service delivery.

Step Nine: Dissemination and Sharing

The recorded songs, which were integral to the research findings, were shared with adolescent participants through a free-to-download digital album. This platform included both Arabic and English lyrics, along with participants' artwork. In Lebanon and Türkiye, SCI-ME staff reportedly conducted follow-up workshops, in which adolescents revisited the songs, reflected on the creative process, and explored potential future actions. These developments were shared with me informally and took place outside the formal research period and therefore were not part of the project's documented outcomes. At a regional level, SCI-ME had also intended to produce an adolescent-friendly version of the report in the form of a graphic novel. However, this initiative was disrupted due to staffing changes and the redirection of resources following the Russian invasion of Ukraine in early 2022. These shifting circumstances made it difficult to assess the longer-term influence of the project in terms of amplifying adolescent voices, ensuring their perspectives reached key decision-makers, or tracking the broader uptake of the findings.[7]

Strengths and Limitations of Participatory Songwriting Research Methodology

The study demonstrates how participatory songwriting can function as an arts-based research method to contribute to developmental evaluation. It provides a relational and non-extractive approach to learning about participants' perspectives. Unlike approaches that extract information without providing reciprocal benefits, this method invites adolescents to share their experiences through storytelling and collective creative expression, activities that often have inherent value for the participants. The collaborative process of crafting individual narratives into a shared song fosters connections among participants and between participants

[7] If I were to undertake a similar project again, I would include in the initial bid and budget proposal additional adolescent-friendly outputs beyond the album, and tools (e.g. workshop plans) to support follow-up by local staff.

and researchers. This relational aspect not only enriches the data gathered but also provides a meaningful, engaging experience for the adolescents involved. The non-extractive nature of the method is evident in the tangible outputs—original songs—that hold meaning for the participants beyond the research context. These songs represent shareable, concise research communication outputs that can potentially reach wider audiences, further amplifying the adolescents' voices. From the perspective of SCI-ME, the participatory songwriting method produced salient and actionable findings, supported through evocative first-person narratives and the systematic approach to data generation and analysis across the 11 sites. Songwriting also offered developmental benefits for staff, building their capacity to further explore arts-based research methods in their ongoing monitoring and evaluation work. Overall, participatory songwriting's generation of rich narrative data and shared meaning-making align effectively with the learning and adaptation goals of developmental evaluation.

Despite its affordances, there are potential limitations to consider. The multifaceted role of the songwriting facilitator is central to the method's effectiveness. Creating an environment in which adolescents feel safe expressing themselves creatively and emotionally and having the capacity to hold and maintain that space when emotions arise, is critical. Effective music facilitation is a specialised skill, requiring knowledge of music leadership, group dynamics, and critical engagement with the power dynamics of creative work. For organisations seeking to use this method, partnering with local music educators, therapists or community artists with group songwriting experience could help build this capacity. However, in humanitarian settings, arts-based activities are frequently viewed as non-essential, with resources instead channelled towards urgent survival needs. This can make it challenging to locate and engage suitable creative collaborators. A sustainable long-term approach could involve organisations investing in developing the musical aspirations of the young people from the communities they serve, independent of specific research agendas. This strategy could nurture local talent, creating a pool of potential songwriting facilitators for future research and community-based creative projects.

There are also ethical complexities around collective ownership of the creative outputs. While co-creating songs can be an empowering experience, it raises questions about who owns that artistic work and how its usage will be determined. Developing clear consent protocols that are revisited iteratively and ensuring project sponsors' commitment to creative and editorial freedom are essential. A related challenge is the potential for power dynamics to unduly influence participants' creative expressions. In one of the girls' songwriting workshops in Jordan, the participants wanted to write about "revolutionary goals". A local staff member urged them to use a less charged word, perhaps mindful of the real risks in their context, or uncomfortable with the idea of girls as revolutionaries. The girls held their resolve and were supported in their word choice by Ameen, but the episode illustrated how easily existing power dynamics could compromise participants' intended messages.

Lastly, there is a need to anticipate the inherent emergence and messiness of creative processes in participatory arts-based research. This requires willingness to navigate ambiguity and flexibility to "follow the 'story' that is told by the research process itself" (Collier and Perry 2021, 87). Thus, the choice of participatory songwriting as a research methodology needs to consider alignment of intention, available resources, institutional support, and critical reflexivity. When thoughtfully implemented, however, this approach can amplify adolescents' voices in ways that encourage decision-makers and stakeholders to meaningfully listen, consider and potentially act upon, the perspectives shared by young people.

Conclusion

In this chapter, I've explored how participatory songwriting can be used in research that centres voice and aims to engage adolescent participants as co-producers of knowledge. Through the examination of a multi-country study with adolescents affected by war, violence, and displacement, I have shown how this approach shows promise in fulfilling these aims while also addressing the dual obligations set forth in Article 12 of the United Nations Convention on the Rights of the Child (UNCRC): the free expression of views and the necessity of listening and giving due weight to what is expressed.

The participatory songwriting methodology presented here offers a relational and non-extractive approach for engaging adolescents in humanitarian research and evaluation, particularly research focused on learning, adaptation, and programme development. In its integration of arts-based practices with qualitative inquiry, the methodology generated rich narratives data about adolescent experiences of voice and voicelessness while fostering youth participation throughout the research process. The collaborative songwriting activities positioned young people as co-creators and analysts, challenging adult-centric power dynamics in research and development action and shifting the emphasis from vulnerability to adolescents' resilience and creativity. This approach produced valuable research insights and created meaningful, tangible outputs that held value for participants beyond the research context. But to realise its potential, researchers, and organisations must embrace the unpredictability of creative processes, identify or invest in suitably skilled facilitators, loosen traditional hierarchies of control, and foreground young people's agency throughout the research and creative journey.

Participatory songwriting thus offers researchers and evaluators an artful tool to support responsive programme development, aligning with goals of facilitating learning and adaptation in complex contexts. Its capacity to unlock nuanced socio-emotional insights makes it an intriguing alternative for those aiming to centre youth perspectives and generate fresh insights and outputs to inform ongoing programme adjustments. While researchers cannot guarantee that adolescents' voices will be acted upon, this method creates opportunities for their perspectives to be framed, heard, and considered in urgent, compelling, and accessible ways, supporting the adaptive ethos of developmental evaluation.

Acknowledgment Heartfelt thanks are extended to Dr Louise Godwin for her work on the original research project and review of literature for this chapter and to musician Ameen Mokdad for his artistry, data gathering, and skilled facilitation in transforming stories into songs. Thanks to Natalia Tapies (Save the Children International) for her insights and feedback throughout the project, to the adolescent participants in Lebanon, Jordan, and Turkey for sharing their experiences of voice so generously, and to the SCI-ME staff who participated in the workshops as co-facilitators and note-takers, supporting the development of the method.

References

Bolger, Lucy. 2015. Being a player: Understanding collaboration in participatory music projects with communities supporting marginalised young people. *Qualitative Inquiries in Music Therapy* 10 (3):77–126.

Boydell, Katherine M., Michael Hodgins, Brenda M. Gladstone, Elaine Stasiulis, Geroge Belliveau, Hoi Cheu, Pia Kontos, and Janet Parsons. 2016. Arts-based health research and academic legitimacy: transcending hegemonic conventions. *Qualitative Research* 16 (6):681–700. https://doi.org/10.1177/1468794116630040.

Bronfenbrenner, Urie. 1977. "Toward an experimental ecology of human development." *American Psychologist* 32 (7):513–531.

Cavarero, Adriana. 2005. *For more than one voice: Towards a philosophy of vocal expression*. Trans. P.A. Kottman. Stanford, CA: Stanford University Press.

Coemans, Sara, and Karin Hannes. 2017. Researchers under the spell of the arts: Two decades of using arts-based methods in community-based inquiry with vulnerable populations. *Educational Research Review* 22:34–49. https://doi.org/10.1016/j.edurev.2017.08.003.

Collier, Diane R., and Mia Perry. 2021. Imagining research together and working across divides: Arts-informed research about young people's (post) digital lives. *Qualitative Research* 23 (1):72–91. https://doi.org/10.1177/14687941211010029.

Couldry, Nick. 2010. *Why voice matters: Culture and politics after neoliberalism*. London: SAGE Publications.

de Quadros, Andre, and Emilie Amrein. 2022. *Empowering song: Music education from the margins*. New York: Routledge.

Fairchild, Rebecca, and Katrina Skewes McFerran. 2019. "Music is everything": Using collaborative group songwriting as an arts-based method with children experiencing homelessness and family violence. *Nordic Journal of Music Therapy* 28 (2):88–107. https://doi.org/10.1080/08098131.2018.1509106.

Freire, Paolo. 2000/1970. *Pedagogy of the Oppressed*. Trans. M.B. Ramos. New York: Bloomsbury.

Green, Amber, and Myriam Denov. 2019. Mask-making and drawing as method: Arts-based approaches to data collection with war-affected children. *International Journal of Qualitative Methods* 18:1–13. https://doi.org/10.1177/1609406919832479.

Jones, Nicola, Kate Pincock, and Bassam Abu Hamad, eds. 2021. *Adolescents in humanitarian crisis: Displacement, gender and social inequalities*. Abingdon, Oxon.: Routledge.

Juffermans, Kasper, and Jef Van der Aa. 2013. Introduction to the Special Issue: Analyzing coice in educational discourses. *Anthropology & Education Quarterly* 44 (2):112–123. https://doi.org/10.1111/aeq.12010.

Leavy, Patricia. 2020. *Method meets art: Arts-based research practice*. 3rd ed. New York: Guildford Press.

Mason, Claire. 2019. *I wish tomorrow will not come: Adolescents and the impact of conflict on their experiences*. Amman: Save the Children Regional Office in the Middle East and Eastern Europe. https://resourcecentre.savethechildren.net/document/i-wish-tomorrow-will-not-come-adolescents-and-impact-conflict-their-experiences/. Accessed 13 May 2025.

Nguyen, Xuan Thuy, Marnina Gonick, and Tuyen Bui. 2021. Engaging girls with disabilities through cellphilming: Reflections on participatory visual research as a means of countering violence in the Global South. *Childhood* 28 (3):380–394. https://doi.org/10.1177/09075682211020067.

Patton, Michael Quinn. 2011. *Developmental evaluation: Applying complexity concepts to enhance innovation and use*. New York: Guilford Press.

Pavarini, Gabriela, Lindsay M. Smith, Nicola Shaughnessy, Anna Mankee-Williams, Josita Kavitha Thirumalai, Natalie Russell, and Kamaldeep Bhui. 2021. Ethical issues in participatory arts methods for young people with adverse childhood experiences. *Health Expectations* 24 (5):1557–1569. https://doi.org/10.1111/hex.13314.

Singh, Neha S., Jocelyn DeJong, Kimberley Popple, Chi-Chi Undie, Rozane El Masri, Ritah Bakesiima, Mariana Calderon-Jaramillo, Ellen Peprah, Saha Naseri, Nadine Cornier, and Karl Blanchet. 2023. Adolescent wellbeing in humanitarian and fragile settings: Moving beyond rhetoric. *British Medical Journal* 380:e068280. https://doi.org/10.1136/bmj-2021-068280.

United Nations. 1989. Convention on the rights of the child. United Nations Treaty Series, vol. 1577, no. 27531. New York: United Nations.

Ware, Vicki-Ann. 2022. Metaphor in conflict transformation: Using arts to shift perspectives and build empathy. *The European Journal of Development Research,* 35:914–937. https://doi.org/10.1057/s41287-022-00546-w.

Ware, Vicki-Ann, Kirsten Sadeghi-Yekta, Tim Prentki, and Wasim al Kurdi. 2025. "Artful development: Arts as research method?" In *Arts-based research in global development: Peforming knowledge*, ed. Vicki-Ann Ware, Kirsten Sadeghi-Yekta, Tim Prentki and Wasim al Kurdi, 3–28. Abingdon, Oxon.: Routledge.

PART IV

Arts as Evaluative Practices

CHAPTER 11

Contested Zones: Circus Science Collaboration on Issues of Australian Ecologies

Linda Hassall and Natalie Lazaroo

Introduction

We are living in a world where human impact on more-than-human nature[1] and species is becoming commonplace, and the dominant role humans have in shaping and transforming natural ecologies is driven by circumstances such as land-use developments, including land appropriation for industry and human mobility needs. The outcomes of human impact on our natural ecologies are often detrimental to the ecosystems

[1] In this paper, this term is used to remind that the non-human world including animals, plants, and ecosystems world not only exists but has causal powers and capacities of its own that can be disrupted by human society.

L. Hassall (✉) · N. Lazaroo
Griffith University, Brisbane, QLD, Australia
e-mail: l.hassall@griffith.edu.au

N. Lazaroo
e-mail: n.lazaroo@griffith.edu.au

M. Mullen et al. (eds.), *Artful Evaluation for Creative Health and Wellbeing*, New Directions in Cultural Policy Research,
https://doi.org/10.1007/978-3-032-17063-7_11

involved and include biodiversity loss (Dirzo et al. 2014), desertification (Reynolds et al. 2007; D'Ordorico et al. 2013), and degradation of coastal ecosystems (Barbier et al. 2008). There is no doubt that as the effects of climate change and corresponding human, industrial, and material interventions on the country increase, our unique more-than-human ecologies are experiencing significant change (Hassall 2021). While traditionally scientists and scientific scholars have had the unenviable role of communicating the escalation of climate and ecological challenges from primarily quantitative perspectives, artistic and scholarly collaborations, as discussed in this chapter, suggest that it is prejudicial to assume it is the sole responsibility of science to inform and educate communities with this information. This is particularly important when "problematic science communication" acts as a barrier to public attitudes and behaviour on climate change in countries like Australia (Tranter et al. 2023).

In response to escalating global and climate related emergencies and ever-increasing industrial activities, some Australian theatre-makers are using theatre and performance methods to explore how ecological deterioration is affecting more-than-human species and more-than-human nature in specific sites of disruption. While key examples of scholarship support sustainable theatre making with specific focus on technical and design processes (Hassall and Rowan 2019; Beer 2021; Hassall et al. 2023), what is particularly exciting about fostering ecological communication through creative methods and theatrical performance is the slow but emerging trend in collaborations between theatre practitioners and scientists and/or scholars.

Science-theatre collaborations are on the rise as organisations across the globe, such as Julie's Bicycle and The Eden Project (UK), Climate Change Theatre Action, (USA/Canada), and CLIMARTE (Australia) acknowledge the benefits of such relationships in mobilising the arts to act on the climate and the ecological crisis. While many international organisations are facilitating such collaborative processes, the "dual resonance" (Roberts 2015) between scholars/scientists and artists is somewhat under-realised in Australia. Dual resonance requires theatre-makers and artists specifically to consider emotional reaction and scholarly information as equally significant in ethically communicating the scientific narrative.

The collaboration discussed here, Climatescape, attempted this dual resonance, uniting practice-led performance researchers, social justice researchers, social scientists, and circus artists to challenge the boundaries between contemporary performance making and social science discourse to engage communities beyond the academic or scientific. Circus as the predominant means of methodological investigation, empowered, advocated, and activated a space for artists, researchers, and migratory specialists to meet and to explore significant challenges in unique and embodied ways to offer the science an alternative way of knowing and sharing. The project was initiated from phenomenological, environmental, and ethical experiences of human-industrial relationships with the more-than-human world, in relation to migration disruptions of more-than-human species in the ecologically unique Moreton Bay wetlands, Queensland, Australia. This unique collaboration specifically explored how industrial and human mobility expansion is detrimental to the feeding and nesting behaviours of a critically endangered Australian bird species: the Far Eastern Curlew (herein referred to as Curlew). Through circus-led exploration we adapted Dr. Kaya Barry and Dr. Samid Suliman's (2021, 2023) social science research about contested mobility developments and migratory challenges in Moreton Bay and, in doing so, united their climate migration expertise with performance (theatre and drama) researchers, and artists from Vulcana Circus (Brisbane). The research explored how creative adaptation of academic writing can be enacted through circus methods to communicate the impact of human interventions in the contested development sites of Pinkenba, the Brisbane Airport, and the Brisbane Cruise Terminal. Drs Barry and Suliman were also active participants in the creative development process,[2] and collaborated with the practitioners and artists on how circus methodologies could narrate the impact of human interventions on more-than-human species.

Throughout, we were unsure what values we hoped to enact successfully in the work because we knew that our creative exploratory endeavours—a process of embodiment and imagination—would not provide any immediate agency change in habitat experience for the Curlews in the region. Further, we could not realistically attribute agency over or ownership of habitat to a more-than-human species through our human-driven response about the implications resounding from human disruptions to habitat. Evaluation challenges were explicit within this process, which

[2] Samid Suliman was also involved as a performer, activating his multiple voices as a social scientist in the dramaturgical translation process as a performer, narrator, researcher, and scholar. Kaya Barry documented the process through film and photography.

consisted of a series of creative development workshops with Vulcana circus artists.

Why Circus?

Many questions arose in framing the project, not only from Hassall's personal creative-research imaginings but from the collaborative team more broadly. *Why circus? How does circus depart from other artistic representations such as more traditional narrative storytelling methods?* For Hassall, in the very early stages of framing the project, she was drawn to the potential of adopting circus methodologies, especially aerial methods, to explore the more-than-human avian themes within Barry and Suliman's work. In circus performances, the bodies seem to want to accomplish the impossible and break limits, seeking balance in moments of extreme instability (de Leles and de Camargo 2022, 2), and the relationship between these moments of impossibility and instability and the exacerbated circumstances of the Curlew were evident. As described by de Leles and de Camargo:

> [Circus] bodies seem to fly and/or float on a trapeze, on a rope, or through acrobatic jumps on the ground, searching for, ignoring, or even overcoming the force of gravity, risking their lives, as if nature might finally come under control, in an instant of time…There is an attempt to randomly fling themselves into the air [or] throw an unimaginable quantity and/or quality of objects. (2022, 2)

We asked ourselves what an unimaginable quantity of human objects might mean from the more-than-human perspective, i.e., things such as planes, cruise ships, fishing boats, heavy machinery, industrial developments, jet skis, litter, and sewerage detritus. *What does this look like? Feel like? How might this be embodied to show disruption to the natural ecologies of place? How could the circus artists explore these questions to express the associated complexities of the environmental and ecological challenges these objects posed?* Such provocations suggest Climatescape contributes to what Australian National University (ANU) describes as the "fascinating and innovative negotiation taking place in contemporary circus—one that transcends the boundaries of traditional performance art to engage with the complexities of the Anthropocene" (2024, n.p.). As a form of environmental circus, Climatescape explored knowledge of the environment through embodied methods in order to supersede the human-centric experience, thereby "acknowledg[ing] the interconnectedness of all living beings and the environment" (ANU 2024, n.p.). As the project was about the process and there was not going to be a production, our focus was on experimentation and exploration. Circus was the means of communicating more-than-human challenges and while it is impossible to assume value against more-than-human criteria, we attempted "epistemic humility" (Bailey 2024, n.p.) by creating space to imagine what might be of value to the migratory birds. We were working reflexively in action, responding to content from floor and arial explorations, and through experimental embodied applications of circus and physical technique. Stimulus material was continually shifting and developing in the workshop process in responses to embodied evocations of content. As such, discussing evaluation is somewhat problematised from the outset as the eco-creative framework concerned more-than-human challenges faced by a more-than-human species as the focus of the inquiry. We did, however, question the process throughout. *Could circus raise awareness about the migratory challenges experienced by more-than-human species in the region? What would be the value for a public audience? What would be the cultural value of this as a fully-fledged production? Does an interdisciplinary project such as this contain academic and artistic value?* With these questions and uncertainties in mind, we embarked on the creative development process.

The process began with Hassall analysing and adapting the scholarly texts into dramatic form, discussed herein as dramaturgical transformation.[3] Initially, excerpts or "contextualised bites" from Barry and Suliman's (2021) article were dramaturgically transformed into performance script, for example:

> Welcome to the shores of Moreton Bay.
> Meanjin.
> To the mouth of the Brisbane River.
> Maiwar.
> To the largest airport in the nation.

[3] This is one of Hassall's terms for taking excerpts of academic writing and transforming that excerpt into a poetic or dramatised re-articulation of the scholarly content to suit purpose of artistic process aims.

BNE.[4]
Moving 23.8 million people.
Each year.
A significant Cargo Hub.
In the Asia Pacific region.
A transit hub for ever expanding.
Human activity.
Land of the Quandamooka People. (Hassall's 2023 adaptation of Barry and Suliman 2021)

The Moreton Bay region that provoked the initial scholarly and later artistic exploration is situated on the East Asian-Australasian Flyway (EAAF), a migratory path which spans 18 countries and carries over 50 million birds each year. Zones of the flyway are exposed to significant, rapid and increasing economic industrial development and consequently many waterbird populations in this flyway are threatened or in decline (Barry and Suliman 2023, 513–532). Barry and Suliman note that "[k]ey sites that make up the Flyway are established and prolific hubs for [these] nonhuman mobilities, yet encroaching land reclamation practices are resulting in considerable avian population declines" (2023, 513).

The Curlew flies over 30,000 kilometres per year and "is a critically endangered migratory shorebird, whose global population has rapidly declined by up to 80%" over the last 30 years (Lilleyman et al. 2020, 1). Loss of intertidal habitat across its flyway has been a significant cause of this decline. The collaborators traversed the borders between determining scholarly knowledge of creative inquiry and artistic and embodied practice, exploring alternative ways of sharing the challenges associated with one native migratory species. Artistic judgement and evaluation considerations were not preconceived but developed as collaborative interactions between the scholarship, the dramaturgical reimaging, the individual skills of the artists, methods explored for embodied narration (Heinich 2012). The circus methods applied were primarily physical expressions and the researchers collaborated with the Vulcana performers to ensure their expertise led the investigation in the creative development space.

[4] BNE refers to Brisbane Domestic Airport terminal.

Transformative Dramaturgies

In Climatescape, more-than-human experiences in the Moreton Bay region became a crucial lens through which the circus artists explored and engaged with the migratory challenges and the birds' endangerment. As stated, the first stage in the process was to adapt and transform the scholarly research into contextual bites of performance script—a dramatic re-imagining of the scholarly text that could be explored in a creative workshop space. The script excerpts became provocation for artistic embodiment by the circus team, which included trapeze artist, social justice researcher, and co-author of this chapter, Natalie Lazaroo, sling artist Chloë Callistemon, and acrobat floor artist Sophie Whitecross. This phase included extracting information from the published research that both communicated the migration challenges and significantly supported artistic embodied circus experimentation; Barry and Suliman's (2021, n.p.) article contained the below passage which Hassall identified as encouraging circus exploration:

> All sorts of things wash-up along these shores for our delight: organic, inorganic, microbial. If you look down, we find a duty-free bag, fish scales, sea glass that has been pummelled by the waves, tangled fishing line, and small bits of polystyrene. The ebbs and flows of the tides leave traces of mobility from elsewhere, evidence of an always connected shoreline being composed by ocean currents and trade winds.

The Curlew is at risk of extinction as its habitat on the EAAF disappears more and more each year. What did risk mean in this context in the workshop space for both the subject of the process and for the artists embodying the subject through their circus methods? Elements of risk, both as a behaviour associated with circus performance and as a circumstance experienced by the birds became a driving force in the creative workshop process. For the Curlew, risk was especially associated with human interventions in place. Marine debris such as plastic bags, fishing lines, and polystyrene detritus are human-made products entering the more-than-human marine environment of Moreton Bay, whether by accidental loss or damage, or wilful disposal (Townsend et al. 2024). The above excerpt clearly identified such elements of risk. When first read the passage evoked a theatrical tension between more-than-human nature and the human-affected environment, for example, the rhythmic motion of waves washing various man-made bits and pieces of debris along the shoreline. In the dramaturgical translation from scholarly article to performance script, Hassall anticipated how the structuring of a rhythmic dramaturgy in the transformation process would enable circus artists to explore the ideas from conflicting spaces—aerial and floor positions. The everyday "spectacle" of polluting and ignoring the repercussions of oceanic pollution in our waterways became an accessible scenario for circus exploration, not from the distanced standpoint of scholarly analysis, but as a form of experiential and embodied involvement with circumstances specific to the endangered world. The dramaturgy applied, imagined alternative expressive and experiential ways of knowing to communicate the impacts of human mobility disruptions to migratory pathways, such as marine pollution to identify the dangers faced by birds needing to land and feed:

> On the Shores of Moreton Bay.
> What is that?
> Look Down.
> Duty free bags.
> Polystyrene pebbles.
> Fish scales and.
> Fishing line snaggles.
> Sea glass smooth.
> Tide traces of mobility.
> From elsewhere.
> Delivered on ocean currents.
> and trade winds.
> From elsewhere.
> A shoreline composed, constructed, disrupted.
> Carrying millions…
> Of more-than-humans.
> Along long-haul travel corridors.
> From elsewhere. (Hassall's 2023 adaptation of Barry and Suliman 2021)
> (Fig. 11.1)

The dramaturgy re-imagined the original text with embodied aerial and floor work in mind, techniques applied included acrobatic tumbling and swinging sling work to embody the motion of natural elements such as waves and wind, and the entanglements of "things" washing up on the beach or of objects (such as plastic bags) blowing through the sky with the natural ecologies. Hassall imagined how the circus methods

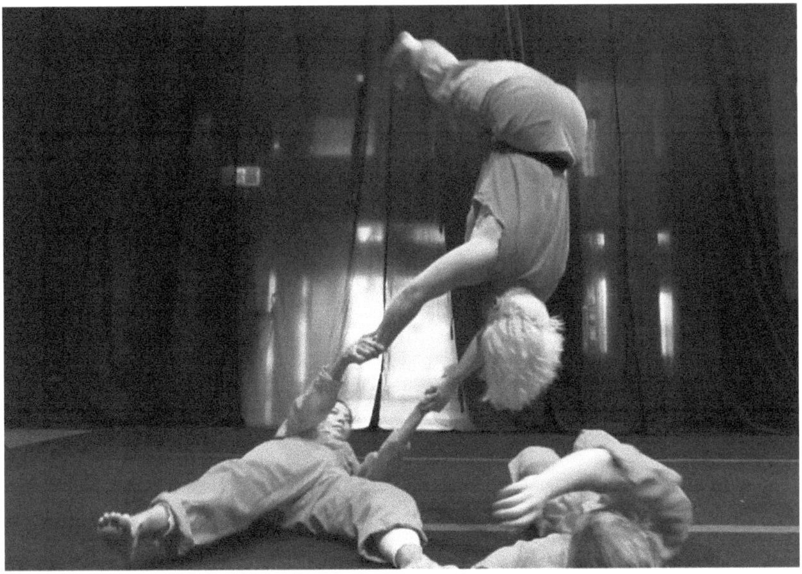

Fig. 11.1 "From Elsewhere." Dr. Natalie Lazaroo and Sophie Whitecross are tumbled by sling artist Chloë Callistemon to represent the washing up of debris on the shores of Moreton Bay. Image by Dr. Kaya Barry (2023)

could both represent entanglement as a physical expression and how this expression of what is essentially the Curlew's inexpressible experiences could be evaluated. *Could an embodied human narrative communicate the more-than-human perspective? Could the methods applied characterise the multiple levels of entanglement between avian experience and human intervention in space and place?* Evaluation, in many ways relied on shifting expressions of values in the workshop and in the arising tensions in the duality of representation in the liminal space between human interventions and more-than-human disruptions in place. Our curiosity, or our hunger for understanding the more-than human experience, spurned creativity—our acts of turning that understanding into new knowledge—and ensured we approached the work with openness (Bailey 2024). As mentioned earlier in this chapter, we worked with a sense of "epistemic humility" (Bailey 2024, n.p.), acknowledging that we would never really capture the Curlew experience despite having a strong desire to learn about the reasons for the possible extinction of an Australian native species.

We conducted site-visits, walking the shores of Pinkenba, observing the tension between the more-than-human species and elements and the non-natural objects in place. On one occasion we conducted an on-site workshop, which for Hassall brought up questions pertaining to how we might be potentially *further* disrupting the site by doing so. The tensions arising in the site—a place of migration and a place of industry (and now a place of performance exploration)—generated theatrical possibilities for how themes of entanglements might be performed. Entanglement as an embodied expression became a provocation for performance and meant an exploration of the relationship between more-than-human species and of depicting the human-generated garbage disrupting the Curlew's migration pathways.

In the studio, the circus team's responses to themes of entanglement were generated from their experiential understanding of the site, their embodied understanding of circus as an art form, and how their techniques could communicate the experiences of the birds in relation to the mobility and industry objects disrupting their migratory pathways. Barry and Suliman (2021) discuss the challenges faced by migratory birds as their habitats are impacted by expanding human mobility hubs and industry. They refer to Latour's (2018) questioning of the scale of humanity and our mobility impacts on the planet and ask for the Curlew: "Where to land?" ...and suggest that... "surely when the winds are howling, the aircraft are in holding patterns, and the king tides are slapping at the remnants of the shoreline, these tiny wading shorebirds must also ponder this question" (2021, 4). The tension between landing and being unable to land is perhaps an invisible one. However, this tension was another driving question within the circus process. For the circus artists, it evoked visible physical expression that depicted behaviours of disruption, confusion, exhaustion, and pain. The following contextual bite communicates the disruption to migration as imagined from the Curlew's perspective:

On the Shores of Moreton Bay.
Where to Land?
Aircraft holding and Winds are howling.
King Tides slap and grab.
Where to land?

Humans run, jump.
Dogs bark.
Jet skis growl.
Boats roar.
Disturbance.
Where to land?
Interruption and disruption.
Where to land?
Rising Sea levels.
Weather wea...THER WEATHER.
War on Space.
No more space.
Where to land?
Exhaustion, Fear,
Where to land?
Where to land.... (Hassall's 2023 adaptation of Barry and Suliman 2021)

The dramaturgical transformation privileged the circus performers' capacity to enact more-than-human disruption through creative embodied experimentation. In such a context, as Kann (2016) suggests, a project of this nature generates a specific circus response to build a dramaturgical performative discourse that took circus technique itself as a starting point for storytelling. With subject and method becoming one, the process implied that evaluation integrated values of the more-than human experience, and therefore, left us questioning how we could do so more effectively in ways that could communicate more-than-human experience and from an eco-justice research perspective, not cause any further disruption to site through our own performative interventions.

Circus as Method

Exploring eco-justice issues through eco-creative practice in this way supports the idea that circus as method has unique advantages for fostering positive change, developing community education and for promoting social and eco-justice advocacy. Because circus primarily relies on physical and visual modes of expression, it can in many ways transcend communication barriers that might be present when only attempting to speak scientific knowledge as spoken dialogue. As Seymour (2018, 10) states, "The body is, of course, central to contemporary circus, whose performers experience a particularly highly tuned engagement with their own embodiment." This collaboration was unique as it scrutinised the tension between embodiment and scholarship to formulate methods that *embodied scholarship*.

In Climatescape, verbal text was incorporated to compliment the embodied experimentation and Suliman took on dual roles of researcher and performer as he joined the performative process as a narrator, responding to the dramaturgically transformed script in collaboration, in situ with the circus artists who physically reacted to both his presence in the space and his narration of the Curlew's migratory experiences. The dual resonance of creating a dramaturgical collision between scholar, circus artist, and performative translation of scholarship complemented the unique embodied communicative nature of the project. As Paul Bouissac (2020, 42) articulates, the visual and embodied representations of meaning through circus acts can be interpreted within the specific contexts of the situations in which they are perceived and can be "framed by the verbal text within which these acts are embedded." Additionally, circus acts—aerial performances in particular—often present both real and perceived risks for the performer (Tait and Levers 2020, 6). Maleval (2020, 53) notes how:

> Circus techniques are an extreme case [i.e., pushing the physical as far as possible]. They mobilize the body in its entirety. The mind cannot disassociate without putting the integrity of the performance at risk. This promotes a shift in the territory of the dramatization.

Circus as method opened up explorations during the process that brought into play an awareness of what, for example, the interrelationships between artists and apparatus such as trapeze or sling[5] could teach us about avian migration patterns. It explored the tension between the physical engagement with the apparatus and the aim of the creative work in communicating the mobility challenges as experienced by the Curlew. Further, "The sensations, possibilities, forms and visuals created in the aerial space" (de Leles and de Camargo 2022, 11), supported themes of disturbance in the birds' migratory flying and landing experiences.

[5] Aerial sling, sometimes referred to as hammock, is similar to silks, in that it is a single piece of fabric that hangs from the ceiling. However, this apparatus has its ends tied at the top of the rigging to form a loop suspended below.

As stated earlier, in the initial stages of the project, the circus artists participated in an analytical process, a process wherein they engaged with the scholarly information for the purpose of gauging their response to narratives presented and how emergent ideas presented themes that might provoke circus experimentation. This was a successful process, generating inspirational content from their expertise as artists who embodied information for the purpose of performative communication. They responded from intuitive, practical, environmental, and ethical positions relating to the human and more-than-human relationships discussed in the articles and significantly drew out stimulus for embodied experimentation.

To initiate the ecological, mobility, and migratory behaviours as circus expression, a series of key provocations were extracted through the team's analysis of the source material and were used to steer the inquiry towards a collaborative and expansive analysis that allowed a diverse range of perspectives to surface and inform the practice-based physical process. Through their responses, two major performative provocations emerged driving the investigation around themes of mobility tension: spatial dynamics and holding patterns of opposition.[6]

Spatial Dynamics

For circus artists, spatial dynamics informs a crucial element of their practice and attends closely to the performance of the contemporary circus body in space and time. As Seymour (2018) discusses, circus challenges normal notions of boundedness and spaces, and therefore has a particular way of mixing chaotic and orderly processes. Some of the first ideas that emerged from their analysis of Barry and Suliman's (2021, 2023) research inspired spatial technique-based provocations for creative investigation:

- *Demarcations* and *boundaries* as relative to human mobility and more-than-human migration e.g., the Brisbane Airport, Port of Brisbane Cruise Terminal, and Pinkenba Industrial sites.
- *Incomprehensible distance*. The Far Eastern Curlew will travel the distance to the moon and back over the course of its lifetime.

[6] Many ideas emerged; however, this chapter only has the capacity for a discussion on two framing ideas within which we worked.

- *Conflicting spatial relationships* between human and more-than-human, earth and air, landing site and flyway. The politics of mobility between human and more-than-human beings in the place.
- *Pursuit of place* and *space*. The increasingly limited sites for the birds to land and feed.
- *Disruption, interruption and restriction* to migratory journey.
- *Collision* and *connection* with human interventions on the flyway.

For the circus performers, the spatial dynamics identified and enacted a relationship with the script as could be perceived in space or in flight, for example, aerial sling and/or trapeze and acrobatic/gymnastic/ground-based investigation. As such theatrical and embodied ideas concerning performance dynamics and energy flow emerged as did thematic questions relating to demarcation, distance, boundaries, more-than-human relationships to space and place. The embodied methods applied structured a physical unification of the thematic threads and enhanced the dual resonance between inter-textual communications—scholarly and dramaturgical—and as such wove together a story that considered theatrical elements of environmental place and psychological space.

Holding Patterns of Opposition

In relation to Climatescape, a holding pattern can be defined as a movement wherein a human or a more-than-human remains in the same state of activity, which can be in oppositions of action or active inaction, wherein they continue to do the same thing while simultaneously waiting for something to happen. Hassall explains this as a sort of Beckett-esque absurdity in performance making (think of the action to wait, to be actively waiting for something to happen as behavioural embodied experience as in *Waiting for Godot* [1954]). The creative expression of what a holding pattern might be, was an idea we also continually returned to as it resonated with the behaviours of the Curlew, but also with the mobility patterns of the continuing arrival of aircraft at BNE airport, which disrupt, interrupt, and challenge mobility harmony for many native species. The conflict in relationships between the more-than-human species, the natural ecology of place, and the constructed human mobility industries, generated several ideas for exploratory behaviours including:

- *Durational activity,* e.g., behaviour resonating the interruptions to landing including infinity patterns, circles, rising and falling, reaching and releasing.
- *Arrival* and *landing* which suggested repetitive patterns of acceleration and stopping, setting down and taking off, reaching for place and being unable to reach it. Importantly, the repetitive patterns evoked the tension of having nowhere to land, i.e., the performative tension of trying to land but not being able to.
- *Stillness* and *motion.* The movement patterns between stillness and motion reflected the *anticipation* of finding balance and equilibrium in the imbalanced ecologies of the region.
- *Disruption, interruption,* and *tranquillity.* The action of being in confusion.
- *Disturbance, chaos,* and *harmony.* Not being able to find comfort, unable to be in harmony with the ecological environment, unable to feed, rest, and nest.
- *Collision* and *connection.* The collision of human materialism and more-than-human nature in BNE and industrial spaces with the more-than-human natural ecology of place.
- *Movement* and *mobility* and the conflicting positions of mobility pertaining to humans and more-than-humans.

The explorations into holding patterns of opposition enabled us to widen the horizons of possible migratory activities through experimenting with ideas on aerial apparatus. The aerial work generated an increased awareness of what it meant to be unable to land, to feed, and to rest, and this understanding was further exacerbated as the circus artists revealed how painful the process was due to how difficult it was to hold these patterns for long periods of time on the apparatus (Fig. 11.2).

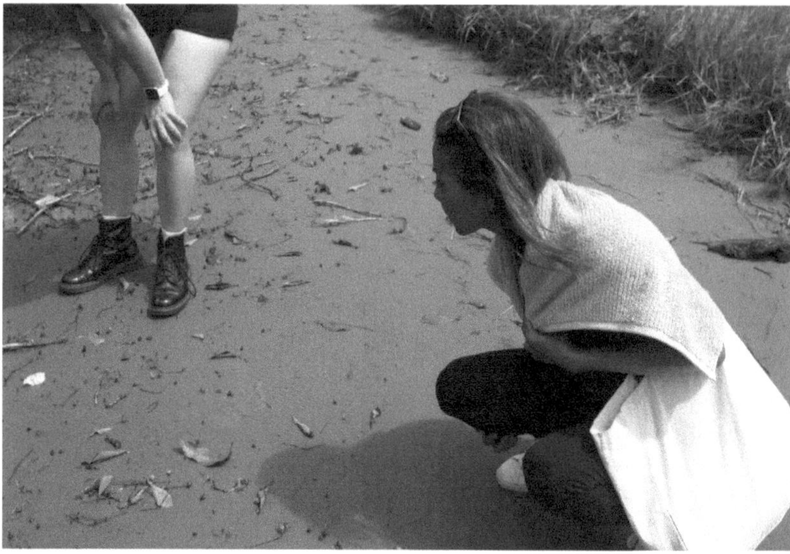

Fig. 11.2 Site visit to Pinkenba. Artist Researcher Dr. Natalie Lazaroo is searching for evidence of where the Curlew has landed. Image by Dr. Kaya Barry (2023)

Conclusion

The Climatescape creative development process was dedicated to exploring and communicating environmental knowledge pertaining to the impact of disappearing habitats on the Curlew through aesthetic embodied investigation. In particular, core elements of circus, including acrobatics, balance, trapeze, sling, and gymnastics became experiences for sharing intangible yet real ecological challenges such as human impact on migratory pathways for the Curlew. On an ironic note, an intergovernmental treaty exists that provides the framework for national action and international cooperation for the conservation and wise use of wetlands and their resources: The Convention on Wetlands of International Importance, commonly referred to as the Ramsar Convention. The treaty aims at protecting species such as the Curlew. The broad aims of the Ramsar Convention are to halt and, where possible, reverse, the worldwide loss of wetlands, and to conserve those that remain through wise use and management (Australian Government 2012). Debates about appropriate land-use in the Pinkenba, Moreton Bay area have significant implications that stretch along the entire EAAF (Barry and Suliman 2021, 1–2). Moreton Bay, Queensland, Australia—the site explored in Climatescape—has five Ramsar sites, but as Barry and Suliman point out:

> Land-use occurring along the shores of Moreton Bay have implications that stretch all along the EEA flyway … it is noteworthy that the Brisbane air and seaport are sandwiched *in between* Ramsar-classified sites… and … the newly developed second runway is in between two designated wetland biodiversity areas. (2023, 525, emphasis in original)

The irony is evident; if the Curlew and other migratory species stick to the *in between* spaces as designated by the Ramsar treaty, they will be protected by governmental treaties that advocate wise land and water use management and support the reversal of wetland loss.

> The Shores of Moreton Bay.
> Home to migratory shorebirds.
> Designated Ramsar sites.
> Local, State, Federal.
> Legislation and Regulation.
> *Protect!*
> *Conserve!*
> Draw a line.
> Draw it on a map.
> Draw it and ensure.
> *Clean and clear separation.*
> *Between protection and extinction!*
> Can you see it?
> There—look.
> That perfectly straight line.
> Between flyway and runway.
> Between runway and wetland.
> Planes on this side.
> Birds on the other!
> Stay this side of the line.
> You will be fine.
> *Clean and clear separation.*
> *Between protection and extinction!* (Hassall's 2023 adaptation of Barry and Suliman 2021)

Evaluation of circus methods to narrate more-than-human species challenges, relied heavily on the expertise of the artists and their ability to enact and embody subjectivity as part of the methodological experience of creative exploration. When evaluating a project of this nature, the word empowerment comes into play on a number of levels. As a team, we felt empowered to continue this work[7] through our new and more comprehensive understanding of the Curlew experience, specifically how the changing world of the EAAF affects the Curlew's interaction within its natural habitat and ecology. Climatescape is an example of embodied scholarship, providing a research framework that empowered us as an interdisciplinary team to unite and investigate the power of circus as an artform, an alternative to communicating social science discourse in more traditional scholarly ways. The methods employed activated a space for artists, researchers, and migratory specialists to meet and to explore significant challenges in unique and embodied ways to offer the science an alternative way of knowing and sharing. The act of creative exploration was empowering as it provided us with confident strategies to tackle the ongoing challenge of "performing" ecological disruption in the Moreton Bay region for more-than-human species. There is no doubt that the creative development process recognised the ability of circus methods to foster awareness, education, and maybe even eventually promote social change within the human and more-than-human relationship. However, in the broader evaluation context, we are still left with many unanswered questions that return to the axiological tension between human and more-than-human conceptions of value. *As human beings—for that is what we are—can we ever successfully perform the inner struggles of the Curlew? Is it possible to embody the Curlew's more-than-human nature to provide insight into its migratory challenges and experiences? Is this project deemed worth pursuing? What outcomes would a fully-fledged production of this nature provide the for the Curlew?* Evaluation in this instance certainly identifies that circus does have a unique ability to enact the problem at hand and generate artistic and academic value (as evidenced by this discussion). However, processes of evaluation were implicit in the creative experimentation that took place at the time in the space and in the

[7] Continuation of this project is funding dependant.

performer's response to stimulus material. Ultimately this creative development experience and experiences framing the creative process were unique to each individual and aligned with their own desired outcomes.

References

Australian Government. 2012. Australia's obligations under the Ramsar Convention: Legislative support for wetlands. Department of Climate Change, Energy, the Environment and Water. Accessed 22 April 2024. https://www.dcceew.gov.au/water/wetlands/publications/australias-obligations-under-ramsar-convention-legislative-support-wetlands-fact-sheet.

Australian National University. 2024. Environmental circus, embodied knowledge of the environment: How can we raise environmental knowledge through performance. Popsicule, Science in Popular Culture and Entertainment Hub. https://popsicule.weblogs.anu.edu.au/environmental-circus/ Accessed 22 May 2024.

Barbier, Edward. B., Evamaria W. Koch, Brian R. Silliman, Sally D. Hacker, Eric Wolanski, Jurgenne Primavera, ... and Denise J. Reed. 2008. Coastal ecosystem-based management with nonlinear ecological functions and values. *Science* 319(5861): 321–323. https://doi.org/10.1126/science.1150349.

Bailey, Fergus. 2024. "ARTD Values: Unpacking the value of creativity." ARTD consultants, News: May 2024. https:www.artd.com.au/news/unpacking-the-value-of-creativity/ Accessed 9 October 2024.

Barry, Kaya, and Samid Suliman. 2021. A tour around the mudflats. E-Flux Architecture. https://www.e-flux.com/architecture/survivance/379365/a-tour-around-the-mudflats/ Accessed 1 August 2023.

Barry, Kaya, and Samid Suliman. 2023. Bordering migratory shorebirds through contested mobility developments. *Geopolitics* 28(2): 513–532. https://doi.org/10.1080/14650045.2022.2027368.

Beckett, Samuel. 1954. Waiting for Godot. New York: Grove Press.

Beer, Tanja. 2021. *Ecosceneography: An introduction to ecological design for performance*. Singapore: Springer Nature.

Bouissac, Paul. 2020. "The staging of actions: Heroes, antiheroes and animal actors. In *The circus studies reader*, eds. Peta Tait and Katie Lavers, 37–49. London: Routledge.

De Leles, Marilia Teodoro and Robson Corrêa de Camargo. 2022. The circus and aerial performances: Simulation of risk and concealment of pain. *Revista Brasileira de Estudos da Presença* 12. Accessed 23 May 24.

D'Odorico, Paulo, Abinash Bhattachan, Kyle F. Davis, Sujith Ravi, and Christiane W. Runyan. 2013. Global desertification: Drivers and feedbacks. *Advances in Water Resources* 51: 326–344. https://doi.org/10.1016/j.advwatres.2012.01.013.

Dirzo, Rodolfo, Hillary S. Young, Mauro Galetti, Gerardo Ceballos, Nick J.B. Isaac, and Ben Collen. 2014. Defaunation in the anthropocene." *Science* 345(6195): 401–406. https://doi.org/10.1126/science.1251817.

Hassall, Linda, Tanja Beer, Natalie Lazaroo, and Saffron Benner. 2023. The Flood Project: Thinking through an applied dramaturgy framework for community regeneration. *Critical Stages/Scènes Critiques 28.* https://www.critical-stages.org/28/the-flood-project-thinking-through-an-applied-dramaturgy-framework-for-community-regeneration/.

Hassall, Linda, and Stephen Rowan. 2019. Greening theatre landscapes: Developing sustainable practice futures in theatre graduates. In *University initiatives in climate change mitigation and adaptation*, eds. Walter Leal Filho, and Rafael Leal-Arcas, 143–158. Springer, Cham. https://doi.org/10.1007/978-3-319-89590-1_9.

Hassall, Linda. 2021. *Theatre of dust: Climate gothic analysis in contemporary Australian performance landscapes*. Singapore: Palgrave Macmillan.

Heinich, N. 2012. Mapping Intermediaries in Contemporary Art according to Pragmatic Sociology. *European Journal of Cultural Studies* 15 6: 695–702. https://doi.org/10.1177/1367549412450634.

Kann, Sebastian. 2016. Taking back the technical: Contemporary circus dramaturgy beyond the logic of mimesis. Masters thesis, Utrecht University. https://studenttheses.uu.nl/handle/20.500.12932/24585?show=full Accessed 21 May 2024.

Latour, Bruno. 2018. Down to earth: Politics in the new climatic regime. Cambridge: Polity.

Lilleyman, Amanda, Bradley Woodworth, Richard Fuller, and Stephen Garnett. 2020. Strategic planning for the far eastern curlew. NESP Threatened Species Recovery Hub Project 5.1.1 final report. Accessed 17 May 2024. http://www.nespthreatenedspecies.edu.au/media/xdvdpzwv/5-1-1-far-eastern-curlew-movements-and-habitat-use-in-australia-findings-factsheet_v2.pdf.

Maleval, Martine. 2020. An epic of new circus (trans. Jane Mullet). In *The circus studies reader*, eds. Peta Tait and Katie Lavers, 50–64. London: Routledge.

Reynolds, James F., D. Mark Stafford Smith, Eric F. Lambin, B.L. Turner, Michael Mortimore, Simon P.J. Batterbury, … and Brian Walker. 2007. Global desertification: Building a science for dryland development. *Science* 316(5826): 847–851. https://doi.org/10.1126/science.1131634.

Roberts, Lisa. 2015. Living data: How arts helps us all understand climate change. *Australian Antarctic Magazine* 28. https://www.antarctica.gov.au/magazine/issue-28-june-2015/arts/living-data-how-art-helps-us-all-understand-climate-change/.

Seymour, Kirsty. D. 2018. Bodies, temporality and spatiality in Australian contemporary circus. PhD diss., Griffith University. https://doi.org/10.25904/1912/1522.

Tait, Peta and Katie Lavers. 2020. Introduction: Circus perspectives, precedents and presents. In *The circus studies reader*, eds. Peta Tait and Katie Lavers, 1–12. London: Routledge.

Townsend, Kathy, Christine Baduel, Vicki Hall, Jennifer Loder, Veronica Matthews, Jochen Mueller, Rachael Nasplezes, ..., and Liesbeth Weijs. 2024. The impact of marine pollutants and marine debris in Moreton Bay. In *Moreton Bay Quandamooka & catchment: Past, present, and future*, eds. Ian R. Tibbetts, Peter C. Rothlisberg, David T. Neil, Tamara A. Homburg, David Brewer, and Angela H. Arthington, 227–244. https://moretonbayfoundation.org/. Accessed 8 April 2024.

Tranter, Bruce, Libby Lester, Kerrie Foxwell-Norton, and Matthew Palmer. 2023. In science we trust? Public trust in Intergovernmental Panel on Climate Change projects and accepting anthropogenic climate change. *Public Understanding of Science* 32(6): 676–818. https://doi.org/10.1177/09636625231165405.

CHAPTER 12

Fleshy Socialities: Evaluative Practices in Theatre, Performance, Health, and Wellbeing

Molly Mullen, Kelly Freebody, Kim Snider, and Elise Sterback

Introduction

All methods for evaluation involve bodies. Even completing an online form is an embodied practice. But while bodies are understood as central to meaning-making and knowledge production in the arts, embodiment

M. Mullen · K. Snider · E. Sterback
Waipapa Taumata Rau, University of Auckland, Auckland, New Zealand
e-mail: m.mullen@auckland.ac.nz

K. Snider
e-mail: ksni229@aucklanduni.ac.nz

E. Sterback
e-mail: elise.sterback@auckland.ac.nz

K. Freebody (✉)
Faculty of Arts and Social Sciences, The University of Sydney, Sydney, NSW, Australia
e-mail: kelly.freebody@sydney.edu.au

M. Mullen et al. (eds.), *Artful Evaluation for Creative Health and Wellbeing*, New Directions in Cultural Policy Research,
https://doi.org/10.1007/978-3-032-17063-7_12

has remained a marginal concern of arts and health evaluation. When bodies are considered in such evaluations, the focus tends to be limited to judging the effects of the project on individual bodies and, often, the underlying concern is with 'fixing' a perceived 'problem.' Rarely are the social relationships and meanings generated through collective embodiment in performance and other arts activities viewed as generative evaluative practices in their own right. This is, in part, a consequence of arts and health being located between or across disciplines and sectors. Not just sectors with different social and practical orientations, but also with different histories, methodologies, and understandings of success. As a result, policy, research, and evaluation in the arts and healthcare conventionally position embodiment and sociality in starkly different ways. Artistic practice, particularly in areas such as drama and dance, often considers embodiment and its collaborative-affective-bodily sociality as core affordances for practice and research and as central to arguments for its purpose, meaning-making, and value. Discourses and practices of health are also deeply concerned with bodies but tend to privilege knowledge *about* bodies, generated by rational, objective cognition. Discourses and practices of health also tend to position bodies either as faulty and problematic, needing to be fixed or managed as part of a policy or healthcare solution. In this chapter, we draw on the ethico-political idea of the social flesh, developed by Chris Beasley and Carol Bacchi (2007), to explore how social embodiment might be taken more seriously in arts, health, and wellbeing evaluation by redirecting attention from the problems with particular, individual bodies to the shared embodied reliance on social space, infrastructure, and resources.

This chapter considers the ways in which arts programmes in healthcare contexts conceptualise the body, and the body's relationship to social spaces. We are concerned with understanding the way evaluation practices in arts, health, and wellbeing contexts often seem to inadvertently emphasise self-reliance and perpetuate a sense of individual responsibility for one's health or ill health. Differing conceptions of the body are, we suggest, one factor in the different ways in which theatre and performance are positioned as health/wellbeing solutions, contributing to a disjunction between how value is understood in the arts and how the arts are evaluated. Finally, we share and discuss two examples of artistic evaluative practices in different settings, which illustrate what evaluation might involve if it was based on the ethos of social flesh. These examples show how arts, health, and wellbeing evaluation might take collective, creative embodiment seriously, and, in doing so, might disrupt hierarchies that are entrenched in what is typically understood to be of value in arts, health, and wellbeing practice.

Social Flesh

Social flesh is a concept developed by poststructural feminist scholars Carol Bacchi and Chris Beasley (2004, 2007, 2012) to provide an 'ethico-political ideal' that challenges the self-reliant, self-interested individualised subject of neoliberalism, or homo-economicus (2007, 280). The ideal liberal citizen, they argue, is imagined as '*having control over* their bodies' and because of this self-control, is considered autonomous and capable of making their own decisions (2007, 291, emphasis in original). This ideal is so ingrained in modern western society that it has become a moral imperative for individuals. Those that do not achieve it are considered, not just un-ideal, but problematic, irrational, and un-well. Under neoliberalism, the freedom of the liberal subject is a freedom to invest in optimising their body's health and wellbeing by choosing and consuming the best products and interventions. Anyone 'considered as controlled by their bodies is seen as needing special surveillance and/or protection,' with such 'help' being devised and provided by suitably rational, autonomous individuals (2007, 291). From this perspective, bodies can either enhance or inhibit the capacity of the individual to make decisions and act with agency in the social space. In proposing social flesh, Bacchi and Beasley aim to (re)connect embodiment and the socio-political in a way that emphasises interdependency, rather than an independence/dependency binary.

At its core, the theory of social flesh first remembers that citizens are embodied and, secondly, that they are a 'body among bodies' (2004, 19). This attends to the social nature of bodily interactions:

> As an ethico-political starting point, 'social flesh' highlights human *embodied* interdependence and in the process configures a new, more transformative social vision. It draws attention to the shared embodied reliance, *mutual* reliance, of people across the globe on social space, infrastructure and resources. (Beasley and Bacchi 2007, 279, emphasis in original)

For Beasley and Bacchi, the emphasis on 'mutual reliance' is intended to equalise or level the social space in a more radical way than theories of trust and care. At the time they were developing the concept of social flesh, many trust and care theories focused on personal virtues, which may result in a more benevolent (trusting, caring) neoliberalism, but not necessarily equitable social relationships. For example, some trust theorists assume that a lack of trust is problematic for society and indicates something is amiss with citizen behaviour. This assumption—that citizens should trust (each other, leaders, governments, and institutions), and if they do not, then should be targeted for intervention—positions trust, like control over one's body, as a moral imperative for 'good citizens.' So, if trust and care are viewed predominantly as individual virtues, unequal, dichotomous social relations (carer/in need of care) are perpetuated. Like more contemporary care theories, social flesh emphasises the way we all give and receive care and are mutually reliant on 'socially generated goods and services' (Casalini 2020, 122). This recognition of embodied interconnection and shared reliance means 'our moral obligations towards others do not come from dependency but from interdependency' (Casalini 2020, 122).

Social flesh is proposed as 'a *political ethic* concerned with existing and future practices' (2007, 286, emphasis in original). It is worth noting in the context of this chapter that the concept of social flesh emerged as a way of analysing and rethinking how governmental practices such as policies conceptualise bodies. However, it has not, to our knowledge, been drawn on to analyse embodied or live processes. While acknowledging that 'writing about' is different to 'working with,' we believe the political ethic that attends to power and care are deeply relevant to both. In this chapter, we are interested in the potential of social flesh as a political ethic for evaluating theatre, health, and wellbeing programmes, many of which have embodiment at their core. We are mindful that in the countries where we live and work, Aotearoa New Zealand, Australia, and Canada, Indigenous understandings of health and wellbeing as relational are recognised and, in some cases, form the foundation of public health and wellbeing frameworks and policies. A full discussion of the extent to which social flesh may or may not align with Indigenous relational understandings is not possible in the limited scope of this chapter. But we do see social flesh as concerned with understanding health and wellbeing as relational and with rethinking enduring health inequities. While social flesh does not offer a framework for evaluation per se, our aim with this chapter is to use social flesh to displace the objectifying, individualising, hierarchical, and problematising approach to bodies that can slip inadvertently into operation when using conventional social impact frameworks.

How Are Theatre and Performance Positioned as Health Solutions?

Globally, the arts are used in health settings in diverse ways. From a general acknowledgement that engagement with the arts (such as going to the theatre) helps people be happier, to targeted and specific interventions such as the use of puppets to explain surgical procedures to children, and everything in-between. Some jurisdictions have well-funded and longstanding programmes, such as Arts on Prescription (Jensen et al. 2024), while other institutions and jurisdictions have a more ad-hoc approach to resourcing arts programmes in health settings such as philanthropically funded theatre programmes that educate children in Uganda about hand-hygiene to combat intestinal worms (e.g., Fleming 2011). While there are few policies that explicitly govern the use of arts in health settings, there are several national and state frameworks that speak to the values and approaches to arts and health around the world, with the focus of this chapter being Australia and Aotearoa New Zealand.

Arts and health frameworks and scholarship tend to position theatre and performance as a solution to/treatment for a perceived health problem, or social problem that may have health implications. This positioning tends to fall under two broad categories:

- **The Generalised Relationship Between Arts and Wellbeing**: This positioning advocates for any and all engagement with the arts—whether it be going to a concert or visiting a gallery—acknowledging that people who experience arts lead to more fulfilling and enjoyable lives. Consuming or participating in the arts inherently fosters connections with others (combating loneliness), provides aesthetic enjoyment (increasing mental wellbeing), and leads to a more active lifestyle (general health). This position drives policy agendas towards a cultural rights approach, focused on increased equity of access to arts as a way to improve community and societal wellbeing (Wreford 2010).
- **The Curative Relationship Between Arts and Health**: This positioning of the arts as a health solution or treatment considers

> the impact of targeted interventions around specific health problems. The arts are used by hospitals, community centres, schools, police, and more to effect change in participants' knowledge and/or behaviour regarding their body or mind—to make children less scared of surgery (Sextou 2023), to teach intravenous drug users about HIV prevention (Cahill 2011) and to improve the lived experience of those with dementia (Dunn et al. 2019). This positioning of arts as intervention drives policy agendas towards impact frameworks, seeking strong evidence of health outcomes from arts interventions (ideally that meet the standards of traditional health evaluation/research).

Beyond frameworks and policy documents, scholarship into applied arts has represented the relationship between arts and health in a similar way. In *Performing Health and Wellbeing*, for example, Katharine Low (2017, 5) differentiates between 'arts in health' and 'arts for health.' Others have differentiated between the understanding of the arts having intrinsic wellbeing benefits, versus instrumentalised health impacts (Wreford 2010; Belfiore 2012). Sandra Gattenhof et al. (2021) rightly argue that the division set up here, between intrinsic value and instrumental impacts may be a false binary, but it continues to contribute to a disjunction between how value is understood in the arts and how the arts are evaluated. This disjunction is of central concern in this chapter.

Notably, policies and framework documents from Australia and Aotearoa New Zealand, such as Australia's National Arts and Health Framework,[1] do not principally focus on the social and health problems or specific participant groups that arts programmes should address. Rather, they focus on the principles of arts in health practice and effective partnerships between sectors. However, most programmes that operate under such policies or frameworks are subject to evaluations that, while drawing on overarching principles, retain a focus on the particulars of demonstrating impact in specific contexts and at an individualised level. Evaluation is key to funding, which is vital for the success of the sector, and funding is typically justified by evidence of impact. Generating evidence for how the arts can be useful to society can also help

[1] https://www.arts.qld.gov.au/images/documents/artsqld/Research/National-Arts-and-Health-Framework-May-2014.pdf.

with advocacy for better resourcing or recognition. The often-precarious place of arts and arts workers locally, nationally, and globally adds to the desire for evaluations and policies that show how useful the arts can be to more mainstream and stable institutions such as health, education, and justice departments. So, even when arts and health policies themselves do not position the arts as a targeted 'cure' for problematic individuals or communities, the way in which theatre, arts, and health programmes are typically funded means that evaluations focus narrowly on what makes them 'useful' to the institutions that pay for the programmes (Balfour 2009; Gattenhof et al. 2021).

One effect of this, we propose, is that a neoliberal ethos and related assumptions about individuals, bodies, and health are inadvertently taken up as the value system against which arts programmes are evaluated. By this, we mean the focus is on solving perceived problems of the individual's misfunctioning or unruly body or mind that inhibit that individual's autonomy, capability, and productivity. So, while the positioning of applied arts as a remedy to health problems is seen by many as a powerful way of understanding why the arts are important and what they can do, we have argued previously that turning the arts into a 'solution' requires us to first conceptualise a 'problem' to solve (Freebody et al. 2019). Often, it is the individuals and communities participating in the arts for health who come to be seen as problematic. They become part of a category that requires, albeit caring and well-intentioned, intervention.

In the next section of this chapter, we present two examples of evaluative practices, which we think illustrate how the ethico-political ideal of social flesh might be translated into theatre and arts practices that focus on concerns for collective wellbeing in particular contexts. We then discuss the ways these examples indicate how social flesh might open up possibilities for understanding and practicing evaluation in ways that value embodied meaning-making and enact more equitable social relations.

Example 1: Becoming Sensory Witnesses by Kim Snider

Bacchi's (2004) concept of social flesh is helpful in LGBTQ+ focused research when examining the materiality of gendered bodies in spaces such as bathrooms. The establishment of gender-neutral bathrooms has been a target of anti-trans backlash, and schools find themselves at the centre of that debate. The notion of bodies as important sources of knowledge was a central concern of my PhD research. It involved students aged 14–18, who used arts-based methods to explore their joyful and challenging experiences of gender and sexuality at school. The project took place at Seton Arts Secondary School, an arts-focused school in Toronto, Canada, with a high population of LGBTQ+ students. In 2015, Seton made two multi stall bathrooms accessible to all students. Student input suggested this model, as it would not require students to 'out' themselves and would allow them to enter the space with allies. Despite support from staff and students, the bathrooms continued to be plagued with graffiti, vandalism, and vaping. Recently, the school removed the mirrors and counter in one bathroom to deter loitering, a decision that my research participants described as 'dehumanising.' The gender-neutral bathrooms were frequently closed for repair, forcing trans students to choose between single-sex bathrooms or no bathroom at all.

In my research, participants shared their experiences of school spaces that felt safe and unsafe, selecting issues to explore through site-specific theatre. They devised scenes for a dramatised 'open house tour' of the school in which we adopted roles as queer and trans middle schoolers eager to learn about the joys and challenges of student life at Seton. This dramatised approach provided a fictional frame for us to move through the school together as we experienced the embodied reality of spaces often hidden from adult view. The following vignette from my research journal describes the participants' site-specific performance of their everyday experiences in the bathrooms.

> We crowd into the main floor bathroom. Scrawled graffiti on yellowed cinder block walls, painted over in a clumsy attempt to conceal their words. Ugly scars where the mirrors were removed. Along the wall, the counter where students often apply makeup is now gone. An unpleasant mix of smells; cherry vape pen, urine, traces of marijuana. Ringo leans against a stall smiling at Ellie, whose legs are propped up on the sink. Their phone is out, suggesting that a phantom third person is in on their conversation. They have written 'out of order' on paper towels and hung them on the stalls and one sink.
>
> Ellie and Ringo converse in short declarative sentences in a variation on the classic 'gibberish' improv game.
>
> Weed. Sex. Alcohol. Vaping. Weed. My parents don't love me and that's why I act out.

> A timid Neil emerges from a stall, manoeuvring around them to wash his hands. They shift and block the way, following him to the doorway. There is a tense standoff. Frightened, Neil escapes out the door. Ringo turns back to Ellie, offhandedly remarking 'who was this bathroom created for anyway?'
>
> The scene ends with an audible reaction from the audience: laughter, groans of recognition. Someone says, 'It's too real.' I ask, 'Who are these people?' gesturing to Ellie and Ringo. 'Cis people. Cis girls and their boyfriends.' Someone says, 'Boys don't come here on their own because it's 'the gay zone.' But they come in with their girlfriends.'

This scene raises the issue of privilege in the bathroom; despite its reputation as a 'gay zone,' straight and cisgender students feel entitled to the space, which can intimidate trans students. Ringo's question about who the space is for suggests a lack of education about the school's gender-neutral bathrooms and the reasons for their existence. On a more sensory level, the performance situates us in the dehumanising atmosphere of the bathroom to witness its unpleasant smells and neglected facilities.

A reflective discussion after the tour suggests more complexity to these issues when students assert that the removal of the mirrors and counter is now making the problem worse.

> Akshay: In fact, it was very welcoming. Because I also would go in there and do their makeup. And it was like, a communal thing. Like I've gone in there where there's a trans person doing makeup next to a cis woman and 'oh, I like your eyeliner,' 'Oh what mascara brand is that?' And it was... just very...it was community, right? And of course there are people in the corner vaping, but like, people are gonna vape no matter what, right? We've seen gender neutral bathrooms with mirrors and gender-neutral bathrooms without mirrors. And one is missing people doing makeup and having fun conversations and neither of them are missing people vaping. So, it was just kind of some solace in the bathroom.

Akshay's description of the mirror and counter as a 'community,' and 'some kind of solace in the bathroom' evokes a space of inter-relationality for cisgender, straight, queer, and trans students. It is an example of social flesh as 'human embodied interconnection,' moving away from atomised notions of dependence to examine the complex ways in which young people rely on and share space (Beasley and Bacchi 2007, 286).

Later in the discussion, Akshay remarks on the usefulness of this area for students of all genders and sexualities, describing it as a 'convergence' of communities:

> Akshay: It was also a connection with cis people because they could use the space for something. They could use the space to fix their hair or do their makeup. It was useful to them, right? They valued the space because they didn't want that space for them to do those things to be taken away. And it was converging, right?

He then describes the ways in which cisgender and trans students resisted the disruptive behaviour of vapers, noting that there were 'numbers' in the bathroom. This commentary draws attention to students' shared reliance on space and the formation of a temporary community that deterred students from monopolising the bathroom. The theatre and subsequent discussion, as evaluative practices, render the corporeal reality of young people's experiences as a possible strategy to combat cisgender privilege in the bathroom. These comments also bring into question the school's framing of the problem as poor behaviour from students; Akshay suggests that some of the students loitering in the bathroom were trying out solutions themselves. Participants' reflections suggest that by framing the problem as the misbehaviour of students, the school has already determined its view of the solution.

In this example, site-specific theatre provided an alternative means to identify and explore issues of space at one secondary school. It transformed us into sensory witnesses, using fictional roles to investigate the problem of the bathrooms. While the bathrooms remained contentious spaces, they may also have held possibilities for 'convergence,' shared interests, and mutual support between cisgender, straight, queer, and trans youth. This dramatic work artfully represented students' shared reliance on social space and explored potential solutions, echoing Casalini's (2020, 122) view that 'our moral obligations towards others do not come from dependency but from interdependency.' As an evaluative approach, this kind of work? may provide young people with agency to 'imagine social alternatives' to issues of safety, health, and wellbeing (Beasley and Bacchi 2007, 280). By touring adults through their worlds, these young people could draw on sensual and visceral forms to communicate 'the problem' as they experienced it. This approach may help to disrupt hierarchies between staff and students and foster dialogue and shared decision making about issues of safety and wellbeing.

Example 2: Moments of Fleshiness by Elise Sterback

The moments shared below are drawn from a workshop in which I playfully invited a group of 15 artists to think evaluatively about the arts 'ecosystem' in their city and their own roles within it. The workshop was part of a larger PhD research project exploring the use of applied theatre methods in the development of cultural policy and how public consultation that informs cultural policy development could be facilitated in more creative and embodied ways. While the arts community is often characterised in economic terms as a sector or an industry, reframing this community as an ecosystem enabled us (me and the participants) to engage with each other from a more holistic perspective. The ecosystem framing was informed by systems theory (Arnold and Wade 2015, Bateson 2000, Bronfenbrenner 1979, Lyle 1985, Orr 1992) and the principles of regenerative development (Gorissen et al. 2024, Mang and Reed 2012), which call for a particular kind of evaluative thinking that attends to the relationships and exchanges within an ecology, and to what might be needed for human and non-human systems to thrive.

Many of the games and activities used in the workshop were inspired by Augusto Boal's (1998) 'Legislative Theatre' approach and its potential for impact in the political sphere, as well as David Diamond's (2007) adaptation of Boal's work using systemic concepts through his 'Theatre for Living' approach. Diamond's work sought to move away from the idea of fixed, hierarchical social relations caught up in an Oppressor/Oppressed binary and programmes that often enact a moral imperative for some groups to take part in a corrective theatre process. Instead, he recognises that whether across different participants in a group, or even internally within an individual, the oppressed and oppressor are always present in the room and that such a boundary has been created by humans. Knowing this, he says, we can then 'use the language of theatre to access the psyche of the larger living community with the hope of transformation in the whole community' (Diamond 2018, 344).

The following narrative examples of moments from the workshop capture how the use of different creative modalities of dance, song, drama, and object play within the workshop enabled such experiences of tapping into a larger psyche through performing together as a microcosm, and thus of the embodied intersubjectivity that is integral to Beasley and Bacchi's (2007) vision of a new ethico-political ethos.

> The people introduce themselves: tossing a ball of bright green wool across their circle whenever they identify something that resonates with their own experience. As the web of wool emerges, they start to silently tug on the ends that they hold, winding the wool around their fingers, exploring the tension. Some people stand, lifting their threads high, while others lie low to the ground. Spaces and shapes form. Shuffling now, wrapping threads around waists, some stepping outwards as others duck under. As movement grows, connections are broken and caught again. They pause. Lowering their threads to the ground, they step back, noticing their web has gone from a circle to become a spikey starfish-like creature.

The web was the first metaphor and tangible experience of interconnection that we explored on the day. The wool materialised the interweaving of relationships that always occurs between people within a round of introductions. At the completion of the circle, one of the participants invited us to dance with the web: exploring and experiencing tension, spaces in-between and the collective shape of our web, our unique essence as a group. This dance allowed us to move beyond verbalising our interconnections and to be present with the dynamics of how a network feels and moves. It was a gentle introduction to moving together, to listening, and responding to each other's bodies. It helped us to focus on the relationships in the room, instead of getting stuck within abstracted discussions of community dynamics, which can happen when we analyse communities at larger scales.

> A landscape has emerged in the room. A ridgeline of blankets and pillows, a rainbow throw for the red-light district. From this ridge flows a river of blue surgical gloves, down into an ocean of polythene blue—an old billboard canvas that fills one end of the room. The sound of trickling water fills the silence as I empty my drink bottle into a bowl at the base of the glove river—activating this sculptured landscape with the presence of a sacred local spring. More offerings are made to the landscape, each person laying down an object that has chosen to journey with them to this hall. An engagement ring, a squishy baseball bat, a leaf, a toy alpaca—each reveals a story about the person who brings it. As the objects find their new homes, new relationships sprout between them—a piece of driftwood

> makes its way back to the sea, a wooden necklace hooked over one of its knotted humps.

Through working with this representation of the local area the group was invited into a dialogue with place. The objects allowed participants to share something of themselves and then play with placing the now symbolic item within new contexts and relationships. In doing so, we explored our shared embodied reliance on this place and geography, acknowledging 'the broad, complex sustenance of life' (Beasley and Bacchi 2007, 293) that we all rely on and perhaps activating a sense of shared responsibility to that environment. The specificity of place was important. Participants reflected on how their personal histories, identities, and practices were intertwined and shaped by the unique qualities of that place.

> The people are dancing now. A fast beat pulses from a portable speaker—it's an ecosystem trance. Each person has adopted a role—they are Producers, Connectors, Providers, and Creators. The ones offering their arms out as support, lifting others up, must be the Enablers. The Disruptors are even more obvious, flinging objects across the space, pushing their way through the dancefloor. Others begin to play with the objects (perhaps inspired by the Disruptors?), wrapping the blankets around their shoulders, folding the ocean into a mountain. They dance across the landscape, reshaping it. As time unfurls and seasons pass, decomposition sets in. The dancers slow, sinking to the floor and a breathy stillness.

The workshop was centred around a collective goal: assessing the health of a system, and what impacted on its health, rather than a focus on individual health or development. Beasley and Bacchi (2007) suggest that an emphasis on mutual reliance helps to equalise the social space. This was reflected in the comments participants made after the workshop, about the lack of 'ego' in the workshop room, in contrast to past experiences of both creative and public engagement. As the facilitator/researcher I was careful to set up my role in the room as one of many needed in this work, allowing space for co-creation and for others to take over the lead of the process or discussion at times. Exploring the different roles that exist within an ecosystem moved us beyond the binaries of being either a giver or receiver, artist or audience, to appreciate the diversity of roles, skills, and perspectives needed within a system. Participants gained various insights into how systems operate, enabling them to: empathise with the roles others play; appreciate where sources of fatigue might exist within a system; or become aware of the need to de-centre certain roles and give more attention to others to support the overall health of the system.

The workshop rehearsed a new way of being together in social space, whether as an arts community exploring their relationships to each other and their place, or a group of citizens imagining new possibilities for their collective future. By bringing an embodied approach to this process the rehearsal started to enact the change it hoped to catalyse. Participants shared how much they appreciated the opportunity to move their bodies—the workshop supported their physical wellbeing, giving them the space to move and rest that they might not have otherwise had. Sometime after the workshops, several participants reported back that they had formed new collaborations with others who had attended, a tangible manifestation of the strengthening of relationships that was inherent in the workshop practices. Participants reflected on the potential of integrating arts funders and policymakers into future workshops, expanding the awareness of the web of interdependency this process helped reveal. Much like Beasley and Bacchi's vision of a breasted lactating Parliament (2012), we might invoke a dancing, sweating Ministry of Culture and Heritage, sensuously exploring its role in the performance of policy, where bureaucrats, politicians, and artists map their shared landscapes, swap roles, and find new metaphors. In this space of intimacy, a new harmony might emerge, generating a 'desirable political imaginary' (Beasley and Bacchi 2012) and a shared hope for the future.

How Might Social Flesh Help with Rethinking Evaluating Arts, Health, and Wellbeing Initiatives?

The concept of social flesh does not lead in any direct way to the use of specific tools, frameworks, or processes for evaluating theatre, health, and wellbeing. Instead, as an ethico-political ideal, it calls for critical and creative approaches to evaluation in arts, health, and wellbeing that take social embodiment seriously. The two examples discussed above are selected to illustrate what we mean by this. The practices presented may not, at first look, appear to be evaluation. But we propose, following through on the political ethic of social flesh, each example shows how collective, embodied creative processes can be, in and of themselves, generative evaluative practices.

Connecting the theory of social flesh to Kim and Elise's participatory, performing arts practices draws attention to the relationship between space and the body. Creating and sharing through the performing arts involved and activated the active interdependence of people's bodies and of bodies with specific places. Petra Kuppers (2022) makes a similar point using social flesh and an ecological perspective to explore the interdependence of bodies, space, materials, environment, and physical forces in community performance. Kuppers does so in a way that is highly attuned to power relationships, for example, she takes social flesh as a concept to consider the ways Indigenous, settler and bi-cultural performances express different experiences of a shared connection to land and to different social aesthetics of citizenship. So, the examples from Kim and Elise show how, with careful facilitation, collective creative processes that are focused on a mutual concern with or inquiry into a shared social space and/or resource might equalise the social hierarchies (e.g. helper/in need of help) around which many arts, health, and wellbeing practice is formed. Together with Kuppers' work, the examples in our chapter also show how working with the performing arts as an evaluative practice based on the political ethic of social flesh might also generate understandings of how different, sometimes inequitable social and spatial relationships are being produced.

In her writing on pedagogies of utopia in applied theatre, Selina Busby (2021), argues for closer attention to the *axiology* of practice, the way in which value is constituted within and shapes practice. Axiological questions, she suggests, are 'questions relating to the concepts of goodness, right conduct, value and obligation' (17). Our discussion above, which considers the intrinsic and extrinsic value in arts and health, is an example of an axiological debate. Without the scrutiny of axiological questions in theatre, health, and wellbeing contexts, we suggest, the alignment of evaluative practices with problematic ethical ideals and value systems, such as neoliberalism, seems more likely. Bacchi and Beasley (2007) call on us to recognise that neoliberalism promotes an ethical ideal of 'atomistic individualism' (281). Neoliberalism also offers a value system that is reductive and hierarchical. Neoliberal processes of valuation function by reducing qualitative details so that almost anything (experiences, processes, objects, emotions, etc.) can be treated as commensurate, or comparable, which then enables exchange and ranking (Kaszynska, 2023,

24). Within and beyond the economy, competition comes to operate 'as a social and cultural process of sifting winners from losers according to scale' (24). Consciously taking up an alternative ethico-political ideal, like social flesh, might be one way of displacing a neoliberal ethos and value system in evaluative practices. In the act of physically being and working together and responding to a particular place, social flesh as a principle calls for evaluation that takes seriously the irreducible, aesthetic, embodied meaning-making of applied theatre and performance. In evaluating theatre and performance, then, social flesh draws attention to the meanings and relationships being expressed and produced through the embodied aesthetics of practice and recognises performance as a practice of social citizenship. It calls for an approach to evaluating arts and health that rejects the body-mind dualism and rejects the privileging of individual rational cognition over collective bodily expression.

Conclusion

Social flesh calls for evaluative practices that strive for non-hierarchical social relations. This presents a challenge to imagine what evaluation in theatre, arts, health, and wellbeing contexts might involve if the practice is not being measured against its success at helping people 'in need' or developing certain individual attributes in those apparently lacking them. One idea offered by the theorising of social flesh is that practice and evaluation of arts in relation to collective health and wellbeing might shift its focus to shared social spaces, infrastructure, and resources on which people are mutually reliant.

We argue that conventional evaluation methods often 'accidently' draw on neoliberal policy proposals that problematise individuals, bodies, and communities. Drawing on ideas of social flesh in our evaluation processes could (re)orient our understanding of the impact of or work in ways that critically attend to embodiment and social caring practices. In each example discussed here, the focus is not on evaluating the effects, or impact, of a creative process on individual bodies or minds, but on using collective theatre and art-making to explore axiological questions and concerns about the social spaces, infrastructure, and resources on which a group is both part of and reliant on for their health and wellbeing. This re-orientation provides not only a potential approach to evaluation for applied theatre practitioners but also one that can be used in the development and enactment of applied theatre work to build a felt sense of connection between participants and with physical, emotional, and social spaces.

References

Arnold, Ross. D., and Jon P. Wade. 2015. A Definition of Systems Thinking: A Systems Approach. *Procedia Computer Science*, 44(C), 669–678. https://doi.org/10.1016/j.procs.2015.03.050.

Bacchi, Carol. 2020. 'WPR and 'Social Flesh' Blog post *carolbacchi.com* posted 30 Aug 2020 https://carolbacchi.com/2020/08/31/wpr-and-social-flesh/. Accessed 14 Aug 2024.

Bacchi, Carol, and Chris Beasley. 2004. Moving beyond care and/or trust: An ethic of social flesh. https://digital.library.adelaide.edu.au/dspace/handle/2440/28327. Accessed 1 March 2024.

Balfour, Michael. 2009. The politics of intention: looking for a theatre of little changes. *Research in Drama Education* 14, 3: 347–359. https://doi.org/10.1080/13569780903072125.

Bateson, Gregory. 2000. *Steps to an ecology of mind: Collected essays in anthropology, psychiatry, evolution, and epistemology*. University of Chicago Press.

Beasley, Chris, and Carol Bacchi. 2007. Beyond trust, care and generosity—towards an ethic of 'social flesh'. *Feminist Theory* 8, 3: 279–298.

Beasley, Chris, and Carol Bacchi. 2012. Making politics fleshy: The ethic of social flesh. In *Engaging with Carol Bacchi: Strategic interventions and exchanges*, eds. Angelique Bletsas and Chris Beasley, 99–120. Adelaide: University of Adelaide Press.

Belfiore, Eleonora. 2012. "Defensive instrumentalism" and the legacy of New Labour's cultural policies. *Cultural trends* 21, 2: 03–111.

Boal, Augusto. 1998. *Legislative Theatre: Using Performance to Make Politics*. London: New York: Routledge.

Bronfenbrenner, Urie. 1979. *The Ecology of Human Development: Experiments by Nature and Design*. Massachusetts: Harvard University Press.

Busby, Selina. 2021. *Applied theatre: A pedagogy of utopia*. London: Bloomsbury Methuen Drama.

Cahill, Helen. 2011. Drama as transdisciplinary practice: Using systems thinking tools to generate new stories about HIV. *NJ* 35: 15–33.

Casalini, Brunella. 2020. The nurturing language of care ethics and other related approaches: opposing contemporary neoliberal politics. In *Care ethics, democratic citizenship and the state*, eds. Petr Urban and Lizzie Ward, 117–136. Place: Publisher?

Diamond, David. 2007. *Theatre for Living: The art and science of community-based dialogue*. Victoria, British Columbia: Trafford.

Diamond, David. 2018. Theatre for Living: Searching for (and sometimes finding) many peaces in the transrational darkness. In *Transrational resonances: Echoes to the many peaces, eds.* Josefina Echavarría Alvarez, Daniela Ingruber, and Norbert Koppensteiner, 339–362. New York: Springer International Publishing.

Dunn, Julie, Michael Balfour, and Wendy Moyle. 2019. Quality of life or 'quality moments of life': Considering the impact of relational clowning for people living with dementia. *Research in Drama Education: The Journal of Applied Theatre and Performance* 24: 38–52. https://doi.org/10.1080/13569783.2018.1544889.

Fleming, Fiona M. 2011. *Acting Against Worms.* Evaluation Report https://www.comminit.com/content/acting-against-worms-evaluation-report Accessed 14 August 2024.

Freebody, Kelly, Molly Mullen, Amber Walls, and Peter O'Connor. 2019: Who is Responsible? Neoliberal Discourses of Well-Being in Australia and New Zealand. *NJ.* https://doi.org/10.1080/14452294.2019.1572432.

Gattenhof, Sandra, Donna Hancox, Helen Klaebe, and Sasha Mackay. 2021. *The social impact of creative arts in Australian communities.* New York: Springer. https://doi.org/10.1007/978-981-16-7357-3.

Gorissen, Leen, Karla Bonaldi, Piet Haerens, and Lénia Rato. 2024. Regenerative Development and Design. Report commissioned by the Belgian Federal Public Service for Health, Food Chain Safety and Environment. https://www.health.belgium.be/sites/default/files/uploads/fields/fps health_theme_file/study_regnerativedevelopment.pdf accessed 25 February 2025.

Jensen, Anita, Nicola Holt, Sayaka Honda, and Hilary Bungay. 2024. The impact of arts on prescription on individual health and wellbeing: a systematic review with meta-analysis. *Frontiers in Public Health* 12: 1–19.

Kaszynska, Patrycja. 2023. Value in Design: Neoliberalism versus Pragmatism. *She Ji: The Journal of Design, Economics and Innovation* 9, 1: 21–32. https://doi.org/10.1016/j.sheji.2023.05.001.

Kuppers, Petra. 2022. *Eco Soma: Pain and joy in speculative performance encounters.* Minneapolis: University of Minnesota Press.

Low, Katharine. 2017. Introduction. In *Applied theatre: performing health and wellbeing*, eds. Veronica Baxter and Katherine E. Low, 3–9. London: Bloomsbury Methuen Drama.

Lyle, John Tillman. 1985. *Design for human ecosystems: Landscape, land use, and natural resources.* New York: Van Nostrand Reinhold.

Mang, Pamela, and Bill Reed. 2012. Designing from place: A regenerative framework and methodology. *Building Research and Information* 40, 1: 23–38.

Orr, David. W. 1992. *Ecological literacy: Education and the transition to a postmodern world*. State University of New York Press.
Sextou, Persephone. 2023. *Applied Theatre in Paediatrics. Children, Stories and Synergies of Emotions*. Abingdon: Routledge.
Wreford, Gareth. 2010. The state of arts and health in Australia. *Arts and Health* 2, 1: 8–22.

CHAPTER 13

Conclusion

Rand Hazou, Sarah Woodland, and Molly Mullen

This book contributes new ideas about and practices for evaluation with the aim of shifting the discourse about the value of participatory arts, transforming the methods by which this value is measured and represented, and confidently asserting the values against which artists, practitioners, and participants want their work to be judged. Artful Evaluation, as conceived across the chapters in this book, challenges the ubiquity and dominance of the social impact paradigm, showing how it is possible to evaluate differently both within and beyond it. Each chapter contributes to a more comprehensive understanding of the value of participatory arts, presenting evaluation approaches that consider the social,

R. Hazou (✉)
Massey University, Auckland, New Zealand
e-mail: r.t.hazou@massey.ac.nz

S. Woodland
University of Melbourne, Melbourne, VIC, Australia
e-mail: sarah.woodland@unimelb.edu.au

M. Mullen
University of Auckland, Auckland, New Zealand
e-mail: m.mullen@auckland.ac.nz

M. Mullen et al. (eds.), *Artful Evaluation for Creative Health and Wellbeing*, New Directions in Cultural Policy Research,
https://doi.org/10.1007/978-3-032-17063-7_13

cultural, ecological, and political contexts in which arts initiatives operate, and take the arts seriously as knowledge practices.

As editors, our common backgrounds in applied theatre have informed the way this collection has come together. We share a commitment to theatre as an accessible and inclusive practice that can platform marginalised voices and experiences, provide a meeting place for embodied dialogue between diverse viewpoints, operate as a forum to inform public debate, offer a mechanism to enhance participation and belonging, and as an apparatus to foster creative agency and cultural citizenship. In bringing this collection together, we have made a concerted effort to present the knowledge and expertise of artists working in precarious settings, emerging scholars, and Indigenous researchers. In many chapters, participants in the programmes and projects are also key contributors. Our editorial efforts are also informed by the need to give back to the communities we work with, by ensuring the theatre groups whose staff and members contributed were funded for that work, and by ensuring this practice-based research knowledge is disseminated in a free, open-access format. As such, we hope that this book encapsulates the ideal of transformative praxis, by which meaningful community collaboration and involvement informs research that is conducted with the explicit expectation that it benefits the people with whom we engage. We hope that the knowledge shared in this book will benefit the artists and groups that engage in participatory arts to enhance the wellbeing of their various communities in which they work.

This book was produced at a pivotal moment: multiple strands of thought and practice appear to be converging to inform a more holistic approach to evaluating arts and health in wellbeing. The recognition of social and cultural determinants of health, the authority of lived experience, emphasis on participatory methods and co-design, the innovative potential of interdisciplinary knowledge collaborations, and the conceptualisation of art and creativity as epistemologies all contribute to this emerging paradigm. These approaches foreground the social framing of health, employing the arts to support critical and evaluative thinking about the factors impacting wellbeing. This shift moves health and wellbeing research away from a focus on individual outcomes towards a broader consideration of the types of change being pursued. Importantly, this perspective integrates evaluation into the process itself, building on the same principles and protocols that underpin the practice. Artful evaluation, therefore, draws on the ways of being, doing, and knowing in the arts to shift the focus from evaluation *of* artistic practice to *evaluative artistic practice*. This approach emphasises the embodied value/s that creativity and culture enact, offering a more nuanced, holistic, and potentially transformative way of understanding and assessing the effects of arts-based interventions on health and wellbeing. Artful evaluation, then, suggests evaluation methodologies that are as rich, complex, and meaningful as the artistic practices they seek to understand.

By looking across the contributions in this collection, some principles and characteristics of artful evaluation in our region of the world become apparent:

- **Contextual awareness and contingency**: Artful evaluation proceeds from an informed and critical stance towards the conditions in which artists, practitioners, and participants live and in which they come together to create. Artful evaluation is **reflexively** aware of how it is shaped by, responds to and intervenes in those conditions.
- Many of these chapters show how the **values and principles** from which evaluation proceeds **are carefully and collectively decided upon**, and revisited as conditions and group members change.
- Evaluative practices tend to be **ongoing and/or embedded** within organisational and creative processes, rather than something that is done to them after the fact and from the outside.
- **Relationality:** Most examples in this volume describe communal, relational art-making, and artful evaluation practices, which move away from individualised responsibility for wellbeing and acknowledge the generative potential of making and meaning-making together.
- **Affective and aesthetic engagement** is vital to enhancing meaning and knowing.
- **Embodied knowing** is recognised and activated, in artful evaluation, creative methods can enable people to enact *embodied value/s*.
- **Imagination**: Artful evaluation embraces the idea that the arts as evaluative practices are powerful ways to critically examine the status quo, and to (re)imagine and (re)create other "possible worlds" beyond pre-existing paradigms. In doing so, value/s can be reconceived and the people involved can collectively determine "what matters" in their wellbeing projects and programmes.

- **Playfulness and emergence**: Artistic practice is inherently playful and spontaneous; artful evaluation embraces this and is flexible and responsive to participants' needs and interests, generating novel ideas and expressions that move beyond accepted paradigms and norms.

We acknowledge, however, that these principles and characteristics of artful evaluation are invariably enacted in the context of rapidly shifting global and local influences, challenging us to hold steady in the face of economic, political, and social upheaval. We now turn to the localised contexts of Australia and Aotearoa New Zealand to highlight specific shifts that influence artful evaluation in health and wellbeing.

Shifting Contexts

Since we began editing and collating this book, there have been important shifts in the wider social, cultural, and political context that signal we might be retreating rather than progressing collectively in a holistic valuing of the arts. In 2023, the election of a new conservative coalition government in Aotearoa New Zealand signalled a shift away from wellbeing policy settings, leading one political commentator to note that "the wellbeing budget is dead" (Walters 2024). In November 2024, the Minister for Arts, Culture and Heritage Paul Goldsmith launched "Amplify", New Zealand's new creative and cultural strategy which sets out the government's support for the creative sector through till 2030. Public submissions on the strategy noted the Amplify vision was suitable if applied to highly commercial arts or creative industries, but less relevant to those working in other areas such as cultural heritage and traditional Indigenous art forms. Other submissions raised concern that the new strategy seemed to "overlook wellbeing, social cohesion, cultural identity, community resilience and other outcomes, and alienates those whose work aligns with these areas" (Manatū Taonga 2025, 8). These shifts might signal an entrenchment of neoliberal value of the arts and a potentially reductive rather than holistic appreciation of their affordances.

In Australia, the return of the Labour government for a second term in 2025 provided some hope that there may be a reversal of the previous decade's declining support for the arts (exacerbated by the pandemic). As discussed in the introduction, federal support for and interest in the health and wellbeing benefits of the arts in Australia have begun to emerge, albeit with still limited resourcing. The Labour government has so far neglected to reverse the damaging conservative policy that saw fees for arts and humanities degrees increased by up to 50 per cent. While there are some indications that this policy has not significantly impacted enrolments (Cassidy 2024), it was an ideological blow that also resulted in job losses in higher education, and it will have serious economic impacts on graduates for years to come. In the current climate of Trump's second term, the government is preoccupied with managing the fallout from trade tariffs, attempting to salvage AUKUS (a major arms deal with the UK and the US), and walking a foreign policy tightrope between support for Israel and complicity in genocide. In Australia, the continuation of a Labour government therefore seems to signal a kind of positive attitude or "vibe" towards the arts, rather than any bold vision or meaningful support that might lead to lasting change.

Resisting Artless Disregard

Antonyms for "evaluate" are "disregard" or "ignore". "Evaluate" implies a careful assessment, so its opposite might be seen as a care-less lack of assessment or consideration. Other possible antonyms include neglect, underestimate, or disparage. We argue that we must continue to resist the various forces that seek to undermine artful approaches to health and wellbeing and instrumentalise their evaluation for economic and individualistic ends. It could be argued that the very practices and ethics explored here will become increasingly vital to nurturing our sense of embodied care, communality, and creativity in the face of metacrisis and systems collapse. The contributions in this book give us hope that this resistance is occurring at ground level. In Aotearoa New Zealand, despite the change of government, we have seen a strengthening of cross-sector advocacy around the arts and a continued articulation from within the sector about the holistic value of the arts. In Australia, grassroots practices and sectoral networks continue to be forged and strengthened in response to rapidly increasing and complex needs across a range of communities and social contexts. The more we enact and advocate for these approaches, the more hope we have of shifting the entrenched paradigms for arts evaluation that seem to persist regardless of the shifting contexts in which we operate.

Beyond instrumentalising creativity for a "brave new world" dominated by technology and AI, the arts can return us to our embodied, interconnected place in the vital network of life and liveness. The arts will always remain a measure of society in a broader sense—holding up society to be looked at. They are an expression of social values and a place where those values can be scrutinised and reimagined. Returning to the ideas that opened this book—how we might "measure" a glimmer in the eye, or a spring in the step, or bubbling laughter, playful banter, a friendly glance, or the gradual loosening of fears and inhibitions—if any "method" can begin to approach such intangible affects (and effects) it must surely be artistic—and artful.

References

Cassidy, Caitlin. Students choose arts degrees in droves despite huge rise in fees under Morrison government. The Guardian, 14 April. https://www.theguardian.com/australia-news/2024/apr/14/students-choose-arts-degrees-in-droves-despite-huge-rise-in-fees-under-morrison-government

Manatū Taonga, Ministry for Culture and Heritage. 2025. Amplify—summary of submissions Report, 12 March. https://www.mch.govt.nz/publications/amplify-summary-submissions

Walters, Laura. 2024, 'The Wellbeing Budget is dead', Newsroom, 22 March. https://newsroom.co.nz/2024/03/22/the-wellbeing-budget-is-dead/

Index

A

Aesthetic, 11, 12, 16, 20, 31, 81, 84, 123, 234, 245, 255, 256, 263
Aesthetically, 116
Ageing, 74, 75
Aotearoa New Zealand (Aotearoa NZ), 1–7, 10, 14, 16–18, 31, 44, 51–53, 55, 66, 93–97, 99, 139, 244–246, 264, 265
Applied theatre, 4, 13–15, 35, 95, 158, 251, 255, 256, 262
Arts-based research methodology, 97
Australia, 1–7, 10, 14, 17, 75, 76, 78, 86, 119, 197, 200, 220, 221, 235, 244–246, 264, 265

C

Capitalism/Capitalist, 43, 98, 104, 110
Care
- cultures of, 80
- ethics of, 119, 182
- methodologies of, 82
- networks of, 84

Care ethics, 118
Climate change, 6, 7, 14, 177, 220
Co-design, 13, 14, 125, 159, 191, 262
Co-designed, 84, 97, 105
Co-designing, 138
Collective or community wellbeing, 3
Collective wellbeing, 20, 61, 62, 65, 182, 247
Colonial/colonialism/colonisation, 16, 53, 55, 57, 59, 63–65, 79, 94, 98, 104, 110, 139, 157, 164
Communitas, 76, 77, 82, 85
Community economy(ies), 134, 141
Community wellbeing, 18, 133, 175
COVID-19, 5, 6, 17, 36, 76, 102, 108, 118–120, 200
Creative wellbeing, 15, 116
Cultural value, 199

D

De/anti-colonial, 117
Decolonial, 8, 9, 114

M. Mullen et al. (eds.), *Artful Evaluation for Creative Health and Wellbeing*, New Directions in Cultural Policy Research,
https://doi.org/10.1007/978-3-032-17063-7

Developmental evaluation, 13, 15, 180, 190, 196, 209, 210, 212
Disability justice, 118, 127
Disability performance, 16, 31–33, 35, 44

E
Ecosystem, 3, 14, 34, 35, 42, 58, 144, 146, 147, 180, 181, 219, 220, 251, 253
Elderly, 94
Elders, 74–77, 83, 84, 88, 187
Embodied/embodiment, 5, 12, 14, 16, 19, 20, 114–116, 160, 204, 221–232, 234, 236, 241–244, 247–249, 251–256, 262, 263, 265
Epistemic justice/epistemic injustice, 115 117, 121, 127
Equity, 2, 3, 17, 80, 122, 245
Evaluation, 8–12, 15–20, 31, 33–35, 41, 51, 53, 55, 56, 64, 66, 74, 79, 80, 82, 84, 85, 88, 89, 95, 96, 100–103, 105–107, 110, 114–116, 120, 124, 126, 127, 148, 149, 157–160, 164–170, 173–175, 178–180, 186, 189–191, 195–198, 210, 211, 221, 223, 224, 227, 229, 236, 241, 242, 244, 246, 247, 254, 256, 263–265
Evaluation methods/methodology, 4, 20, 105, 109, 134, 178, 179, 256, 263
Evidence-based, 10

F
First Nations, 12, 14, 15, 197
Fund/funding/funder/funded, 3, 5, 6, 10–12, 15–17, 20, 33, 35, 40, 41, 44, 51, 53, 56–59, 62–66, 79, 80, 95, 101–103, 105, 110, 116, 134–136, 138, 139, 147, 148, 150, 168, 170, 245, 247, 254, 262

G
Gift, 16, 41, 43, 76, 77, 85, 101
Giving, 10, 42, 43, 47, 76, 110

H
Hauora, 2, 53, 160, 161, 175
Health equity, 8, 97
Holistic, 251, 262–264
Holistic wellbeing/holistic health, 52, 53, 136, 137, 144, 145, 150
Home Ground, 17, 97

I
Indigenous, 2, 8–10, 12, 14–16, 51, 53, 58, 94, 95, 97–99, 139, 157, 159, 160, 162, 164, 262, 264
Inequities, 93
Instrumentalise/instrumentalisation, 115, 127, 265

J
Jackson, Adrian, 3, 4, 156
Justice system, 17, 93, 95, 97, 98, 101, 104, 108–110, 117

L
LGBTIQ+, 74–77, 80, 83, 84

M
Māori, 2, 3, 19, 55, 56, 61, 65, 66, 94, 97–101, 103, 139, 144, 157, 159, 160, 162–164, 167

Measure/measurement, 5, 8–10, 12, 17, 53, 59, 62, 79–84, 87, 88, 96, 97, 103, 116, 123, 133, 136, 137, 144, 149, 150, 170, 265, 266
Mental health, 7, 18, 61, 65, 114, 115, 117, 121, 159, 162, 163, 165, 168
Methods of evaluation, 5, 36, 116

P

Pacific Peoples, 16, 17, 55–59, 63, 65
Pandemic, 5–7, 36, 38, 84, 87, 102, 118, 119, 157, 264
Participatory action research, 13
Participatory arts, 1, 3, 9–11, 17, 86, 87, 95, 122, 161, 261, 262
Participatory arts-based research, 198, 211
Participatory evaluation, 136
Participatory methodologies, 17
Participatory methods, 13, 15, 262
Participatory or relational arts, 127
Participatory qualitative research methods, 13
Participatory research methods, 18
Participatory songwriting, 19
Pasifika, 53, 55–58, 60–64, 66
Policy, 5–7, 9, 10, 13, 16, 51, 53, 55, 56, 59–63, 65, 66, 80, 84, 114, 124, 160, 264, 265
Polycultural capital, 53, 54, 57, 61, 62, 65
Precarity, 2, 5, 18, 157
Psychosocial impact, 83

R

Racism, 54, 61, 93, 94, 120
Relational/relationality/relationally, 15, 19, 80, 85, 89, 124, 182, 184, 196, 199, 205, 209–211, 244, 263
Return on investment, 141, 149
  community economies return on investment, 134, 141
  social return on investment, 134

S

Self-determination, 17, 52, 61, 64, 82, 170
Self-determine, 74
Self-determined, 79, 82, 84
Social flesh, 19, 20, 242–244, 247, 249, 254–256
Social impact, 10–13, 245, 261
Social justice, 114, 115, 122, 178, 191, 220, 225
Socially engaged arts, 17, 78, 79, 82, 83, 85, 86, 88, 115, 122
Socially engaged performance art, 76
Songwriting, 199
Strengths-based, 57, 61, 198

T

Te Tiriti o Waitangi, 17, 94, 99
Theatre, 262
Theory of change, ToC, 157–159, 174, 179–183, 185, 186, 189–191
Trauma-informed, 103, 121, 122

Y

Young people, 16, 18, 19, 53, 54, 56, 61, 62, 65, 66, 173, 174, 176–179, 181, 182, 184–187, 190, 191, 196, 198, 199, 210–212, 249, 250

Kolibri 360 GmbH
Ferdinand-Jühlke-Straße 7
99095 Erfurt, Deutschland
produktsicherheit@kolibri360.de